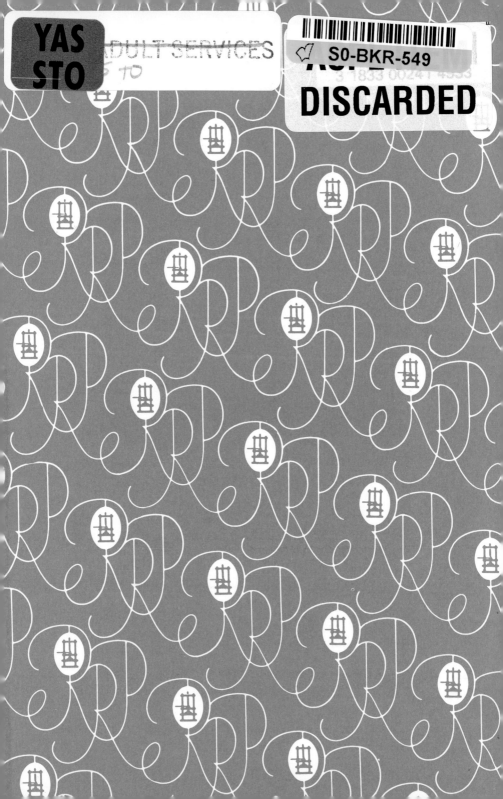

YOUR FUTURE: A GUIDE
FOR THE HANDICAPPED TEENAGER

YOUR FUTURE:
A GUIDE FOR THE
HANDICAPPED TEENAGER

By
S. NORMAN FEINGOLD
and
NORMA R. MILLER

THE ROSEN PUBLISHING GROUP, INC.
New York

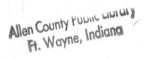

Published in 1981, 1986 by the Rosen Publishing Group
29 East 21st Street, New York City, New York 10010.

Revised Edition 1986

Library of Congress Cataloging in Publication Data

Feingold, S   Norman, 1914–
    Your future.

    (Careers in depth)
    SUMMARY: More than 60 handicapped persons share
their experiences and secrets of successful living in
this guide to developing a career and a life-style.
    1.   Handicapped youth—United States—Life skills
guides—Juvenile literature.   [1.–Physically handicapped.
2.   Mentally handicapped.   3.   Vocational guidance]
I.   Miller, Norma R., joint author.   II.   Title.
HV1569.3.Y68F44   331.5'9'0973   80–21084
ISBN 0–8239–0424–5

Manufactured in the United States of America

This book is dedicated with love and affection to more than sixty handicapped persons who contributed to it, as well as to Marie Feingold and Donald Miller, two significant others who made this dream a reality.

A special debt of gratitude is extended to two nonhandicapped workers, Curtis Iddings, Jr., Virginia Department of Rehabilitative Services, Woodrow Wilson Rehabilitation Center, Steve Bell, ABC Good Morning America, and Keith Roberts of the National Easter Seal Society for Crippled Children and Adults, and to Jo Ann Haseltine, Thomas Lyczks, Fred Mancuso, Birdie Minor, and Clare Jo Schnitz.

HANDICAPPED . . .

At the time of this printing, federal, state, and local funding programs are in rapid transition. For information regarding changes, write to the agencies and organizations listed in this book.

About the Authors

DR. S. NORMAN FEINGOLD is the new President of the National Career and Counseling Services in Rockville, Maryland, and he is in private practice in Washington, D.C. He serves as a vocational consultant to the Social Security Administration, he is a former member of the Accrediting Commission of the National Home Study Council. He is a member and chairman of local and national scholarship committees.

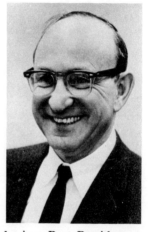

Dr. Feingold received his bachelor's, master's, and doctorate degrees from Indiana, Clark, and Boston universities, respectively. He is a Past President of the American Personnel and Guidance Association. He is a professional member of the National Vocational Guidance Association, of which he is a Past President; a Fellow of the American Psychological Association; and a member of the Massachusetts and Maryland Psychological Associations and the Gerontological Society. He is a licensed psychologist in the District of Columbia, a member of the D.C. Psychological Association, and has served on its Board of Directors. He also holds membership in numerous other professional organizations. A former Executive Director of the Boston Jewish Vocational Service and Work Adjustment Center and Honorary National Director of the B'nai B'rith Career and Counseling Services, he has been a guest professional lecturer at more than 25 universities, a member of the faculty of Boston University School of Education and College of Business Administration, Professorial lecturer in psychology at American University, and Professor of Education at George Washington University.

Dr. Feingold is the author of 30 books, including six volumes of *Scholarships, Fellowships and Loans,* and more than 125 professional articles. He is the past editor of the B'nai B'rith Career and Counseling Services magazine, *Counselor's Information Service.*

An officer during World War II, he served as a psychologist. He is listed in *Who's Who in America.* Dr. Feingold is a member of B'nai B'rith Argo Lodge and the Torch Club, Washington, D.C. He and his wife have four daughters.

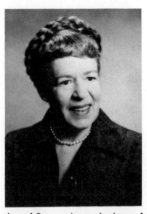

NORMA RENO MILLER is experienced in handling special communications for education, health, trade, and professional associations. She has written career information booklets for the National Coal Association, The American Florists' Association, The National Coatings Institute, and the American Woman's Society of Certified Public Accountants. She has worked for the National Vocational Guidance Association, The National Education Association, and other institutions.

Mrs. Miller has had her own public relations firm, which served the above organizations as well as local chapters of the National Lung Association, the American Cancer Society, and the National Easter Seal Society for Crippled Children and Adults. She received BS and MS degrees in speech and education from the University of Wisconsin. She is currently on the faculty of the Graduate School of the U.S. Department of Agriculture.

She has written many articles and newsletters and a textbook, *Influencing Others Through Persuasive Speaking.*

Mrs. Miller and Dr. Feingold have worked together for many years on various projects.

Contents

Introduction

This book is a practical guide to encourage handicapped young persons who are on the threshold of finding their particular places in the world of work, and who are developing life-styles that will characterize them in their adult lives. It is also about some young and some not so young handicapped persons who have succeeded in making contributions to themselves, their families, and their communities.

Most people's image of "the handicapped" is strongly influenced by seeing an occasional person in a wheelchair or one being led by a Seeing Eye dog. Yet those with such "visible" handicaps are only a small percentage. Who are the handicapped? How many of them are there?

The U.S. Council for the Independent Year of Disabled Persons estimates there are more than 35,000,000 handicapped people of all ages in the United States. This includes those with invisible handicaps such as learning disabilities, deafness, and epilepsy and those sufferers from diseases that may become increasingly and visibly disabling over the years. Examples of the latter are muscular dystrophy, multiple sclerosis, heart disease, and arthritis. In other words, "the handicapped" includes a very wide range of people. Some are severely or even multiply handicapped. Some are only slightly and invisibly handicapped. If you follow this idea far enough, you soon discover that everyone is handicapped in some way. No one is absolutely perfect. Learning to accept, to live with, to compensate for or overcome handicaps is a part of life for everyone.

Who, then, are the 20,000,000 referred to by the President's Committee? The U.S. Department of Health and Human Resources defines a handicapped person as anyone with a physical or mental disability that substantially impairs or restricts one or more of such major life activities as walking, seeing, hearing, speaking, working, or learning.

This book is for all teenagers who may fit any part of that definition. The use of "the handicapped" is a communications convenience, but it can be misleading and inaccurate. There is no one class of handicapped people. Every person is different. Every person has different needs, interests, abilities, goals, and aspirations. A more appropriate term, according to many handicapped persons, is "the disabled." "A handicap is a state of mind. A disability is a physical condition," says Henry Henscheid, who is the Director of Advocacy for the forty-three chapters of the California Easter Seal Society. Henry Henschied was born with cerebral palsy.

The authors of this book define a handicapped person as one whose needs for education, communications, transportation, and living and working facilities differ significantly from the needs of nonhandicapped persons. We shall discuss some of these needs and specific ways in which you, a handicapped teenager, can meet them. With the help of this book, you can begin to plan, right now, for those exciting post-high school years when you will move toward the world of work and more complete self-sufficiency.

More than sixty handicapped persons have contributed to this book by sharing their experiences and providing examples. You will learn their thinking as well as ours on such topics as how to select a career area and how to find and finance needed education or training. There are some tips for landing your first job. A summary of legal rights that apply to both the working and the nonworking parts of your life appears toward the middle of the book. The last few chapters are devoted to your developing life-style. Here again, handicapped persons contribute examples and ideas on independent living, transportation, recreation, sports, and the arts. In the last chapter they share some of their secrets of successful living.

"Don't Tell Me I Can't" is the headline for a story that appeared in the Washington *Post* on August 29, 1978. As you read the story of Jim Brunotte, who is a triple amputee, see how many of his secrets of success you can find. Here is an excerpt from the newspaper story:

Jim Brunotte was always a hell-raiser.

It started in Chicago in 1947 when he came out of his mother's womb a blue baby. At the age of 6 he contracted polio and the doctors told him he'd never walk again.

"This," he said, "is ridiculous." He decided he wanted to walk.

So he walked. They told him the resulting curvature of his spine would prevent him from riding horses again. "Forget it," Brunotte said. He politely told them what they could do with their stethoscopes and sneaked out each weekend to a suburban riding stable.

He rode.

Now at 31, Brunotte has the ribbons and medals on his wall to prove he's a top horseman. Just the other day at his San Luis Obispo County ranch, Brunotte galloped into the sunset on his Morgan charger, Can Can, leaving his 80 gaping guests in the dust.

Brunotte doesn't have any legs. He lost them the same time he lost his left lower arm and his right eye.

In October 1968 Brunotte and an army buddy were making a routine dispatch run down a mile-long road near Bien Hoa, South Vietnam. Their jeep ran over a culvert fixed with an artillery round equivalent to 35 pounds of dynamite.

Brunotte woke up in the hospital disoriented, but ready to go back to his outpost. The nurse told him what had happened. The expression on his face didn't change. He just shook his head and said "Charlie [the Viet Cong] sure does a good job."

He told the nurse he wanted to sit up. She told him he couldn't. "Don't tell me I can't," he said.

And that was the beginning of a new life for Jim Brunotte. From then on he never used the word can't. It's a word he doesn't allow used on his 367-acre Rancho Kumbya, a nonprofit recreation ranch for the handicapped. And if you do say I can't, Brunotte might just swing his body down off his horse and pin you down in the sand until you change your mind.

Jim Brunotte has achieved a rewarding career and an enjoyable life-style. While it may seem that he was pushed into it by circumstances, it never would have happened without his persistence and planning. Later, the story tells of how he gained competence by taking advantage of the Army hospital's special training facilities, then took a job as caretaker on a 3,000-acre ranch, patrolling every day on horseback. He needed planning and persistence in finding and developing his present ranch, and later in finding himself a wife.

In 1979 the whole country recognized Jim Brunotte's achievements when he was named Handicapped American of the Year by the President's Committee on Employment of the Handicapped.

You might be thinking, "This character sounds unbelievable," yet the story is true. Dropping the "I can't" way of thinking from your approach to your career and your life-style is one of the secrets of success for both handicapped and nonhandicapped people. If you tend to think "I can't" about anything but are unable to drop it "cold turkey," a good substitute attitude is "I'll give it a try."

During the next few weeks or months or years, as you develop your career plans and your life-style, try everything you have an opportunity to try. Try things that your reason tells you you may be good at and enjoy doing. You will be surprised how much you learn about yourself. Begin in the very next chapter to lay your plans for your career and for your life-style.

YOUR FUTURE: A GUIDE
FOR THE HANDICAPPED TEENAGER

CHAPTER I

Drawing Up a Winning Game Plan for Your Career

Developing a game plan to reach your objectives is popular these days. It is a concept that is applied to everything from getting a seat in the bus to being accepted by the college of your choice. While *game plan* may be the popular jargon, the development of careful plans to achieve your objectives has always been an important element of success. In this chapter we shall discuss how you can develop a positive career game plan. Its purpose is to lead you to find the best place, and possibly an alternative place, for you in the world of work.

For some this may mean full-time work in one of the professions, trades, or business. For others it may mean part-time work. For still others it may mean careers that can be pursued in sheltered workshops or at home.

A GOOD PLAN IS ONE THAT WORKS

The unfortunate part is that you never know for sure whether a plan will work until you put it to the test. This is usually a long time after you have invested your time in making it, so why plan? Everyone knows someone who just stumbled into an interesting career. Everyone also knows many more people who have given much thought and planning to their careers. They acquired the needed education or training and worked to meet all the qualifications for entry into their chosen field.

The choice is up to you. You can let the stumbler be your role model, and very few stumbles lead to success. Or you can take a positive, intelligent part in finding your way into the most appropriate career for you. The process calls for pulling together much information about yourself that you may already know. You are the number one expert on the subject. It calls for finding the answers to a number of other questions you yourself will raise as you go along. Few people can engage in such self-analysis without gaining some useful insights into themselves.

FROM NOW UNTIL YOUR CAREER—THREE STAGES

During your years of adolescence you will think your way through a number of stages regarding the question of what to do with the rest of your life. The first stage, which we shall call the *research stage,* has to do with deciding a general career area in which you are interested and have ability. The second stage is the *career pursuit* stage. It includes finding and obtaining any needed education or training. This may take from a few weeks to several years, depending on the area in which you are interested. The third stage is the *job acquisition* stage, when you will find your first full-time position in your chosen field.

You may be well along the way in any one of these stages. But for the purposes of this book we shall begin with the first stage and go through all three.

The Research Stage

The objective of the research stage is to find out as much as you can about any career areas you think you may be interested in and be able to enter. There are 30,000 job titles recognized in standard references. Jobs are related to one another in clusters. This means that when you qualify for one job, you also will qualify for other jobs that are closely related in the cluster. They require similar training, skills, and education.

At this point you may have only a few vague ideas about the career areas in which you are interested. Use this initial research time to explore every possibility that occurs to you. Vocational guidance counselors and rehabilitation counselors can be very helpful in finding information on areas in which you are interested. They may also come up with some ideas you never thought of but may appeal to you.

Some ways to find vocational guidance counselors and rehabilitation counselors are listed in the resources section for Chapter II. Also there are sources for information about career areas in general.

The Career Pursuit Stage

The career pursuit stage is the time when you will be acquiring any needed post-high school education or training to qualify you for work in your chosen field. The research stage also continues through this second stage. You will be learning a lot more about your field of work as you study and train for it. Ways to locate the best education or training opportunity and ways to finance them will be discussed in Chapters III and IV.

The Job Acquisition Stage

As you near the end of any post-high school education or training you undertake, you will be thinking increasingly of finding a job in your chosen career. Tips on finding a job are given in Chapter V.

KEYS TO SUCCESS—RESEARCH, PLANNING, SELF-KNOWLEDGE

Making Lists

In all three of the stages mentioned above, thorough research and careful planning are the ways to assure success. One good place to start your planning is to make a lot of lists. Put everything on a list, including questions that come to mind, how-to-do-it questions, career areas you think you may be interested in, questions about the kind of training needed. Your first lists may seem quite jumbled. Don't give up. Study them. Rearrange them and gradually your priorities will appear. For example, you might start by setting down all the thoughts and questions you have on the three stages discussed above. Put down everything you can think of. Don't worry about keeping them in categories. As you study this preliminary list, you will see that some of the items pertain to the research stage, some to the career pursuit stage, and some to the job acquisition stage. At this point you can begin to make three separate, more orderly lists. As you begin your second round of lists, you may wish to rule the paper about two-thirds of the way across. In the left-hand column enter your thoughts and questions. In the right-hand column place any questions or notes of action to be taken opposite the question to which they pertain. Are there letters to be written? Phone calls to be made? Or how can you find out about the item? As your list becomes more specific, you will perceive a pattern of priorities. You can then number the items in the order in which they should be accomplished.

Once you have incorporated all the items from your original list onto one or more specific and better-organized lists, throw away the old list. It can become confusing if you keep it.

Lists, usually a lot of different lists, are the starting point of successful planning. Don't depend upon your memory. Keep a note pad or special career notebook handy and always be ready to note down your thoughts as they occur to you. A plan is an integrated combination of actions designed to gain a specific, predetermined goal. As you begin to refine your lists, you are deciding which steps to take and in what order. You are planning!

One way to make good use of this book would be to develop a master planning list for each chapter. These lists could be the starting place for more specific planning later.

Do You Know Yourself?

To find out about jobs and careers and how to prepare yourself for them, you will need to go to a number of outside sources. In order to find out about yourself, you must depend to a great extent at this stage of your planning on self-analysis. Make a separate list of the things to be considered and questions to be answered, based on what you know about yourself. This list will be different for each person. Here are some questions you can ask yourself to get the list started:

- What abilities, interests, potentials, and personalities make up the real you?
- How bright are you? What is your level of educational achievement?
- Do you like to study, go to school? Do you enjoy reading?
- What tasks are you good at? Writing? Speaking? Math and numbers? Music or art? Or what?
- What values are important to you? Can you define them?
- What do you really enjoy doing? Favorite pastime? Special interest?
- What special skills have you acquired? Circle those in which you have had training.
- In your opinion what are your major achievements?
- How much do you really want to work? Full time? Part time?
- How hard are you willing to work?
- How hard are you willing to work to gain any needed education or training?
- What are your specific health and disability problems? (List those *you* feel need to be considered. List separately any that other people feel may need to be considered.)

As you get into your personal self-knowledge listing project, you will discover other questions and character traits that pertain especially to you. Be sure to include any good character traits. For example, if you have developed good work habits in school, habits that lead you to accomplish your goals with a minimum of wasted effort, put this down. If you have good records for promptness and regular attendance, note these on your list also. As you work on this very personal list, you will be discovering some of the strongest personal qualifications you have to offer future friends, companions, and employers.

BE AN HONEST, FLEXIBLE, AND REALISTIC PLANNER

Honesty

The career game plans you come up with during the next few years will be much more productive if you make it a rule to be honest with yourself. Remember that you don't have to show any part of your plan to anyone unless you want to. Learn to distinguish between your own opinions and how you feel about yourself, and other people's opinions and how you *think* they feel about you. It is more important to sound planning to understand yourself, your own feelings and capacities.

It can also be helpful to understand how and why other people feel the way they do about you. Try hard to look at yourself from another person's point of view and honestly understand why that person evaluates you as he or she does. Talk to people whose judgment you value. Be as objective about your assets and limitations as you possibly can be.

Flexibility

All good plans are flexible. Military personnel include in their planning for a military engagement a contingency plan. This essentially outlines what to do in case things don't go according to the original plan. It is always a good idea to have an alternate plan. You may wish to develop a few alternate ideas for your career, but such contingency plans need not be done in detail. You do, however, need to be flexible in your planning. In the carrying out of any plan, an abrupt change may be called for. Some of the most remarkable examples of flexibility and adaptation have been provided by young accident victims.

Ed Scherer is a paraplegic who works for the Federal Reserve Bank. Since he broke his neck in a diving accident in the early 1970's Ed has achieved his college education plus a master's degree. In his wheelchair he went job-hunting on his own. A few years ago, he was married. That was another great step in developing his game plan for a satisfying life-style. We don't know what career Ed planned before the accident. We do know that he was flexible enough to switch to a career he could handle from his wheelchair.

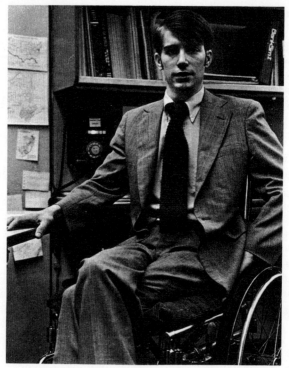

Ed Scherer

Joni Eareckson was paralyzed from the neck down after a diving accident when she was seventeen. She had just graduated from high school, where she was voted "class athlete." An accomplished horsewoman, she had already been accepted by the college of her choice. At first she could not accept the fact that she was paralyzed. She became depressed. She admits, "I think I would have tried to commit suicide if I had had a way." She gave up her plans for college. Her deep faith in God and her own indomitable spirit came more and more to her aid as she began to put her life back together. Today, Joni is a successful writer and artist. She uses a mouth stick instead of her hands. Had she not been flexible and, as she puts it, "come to grips with myself," she could never have achieved these things.[1]

Paul Yeung's story might at first appear to illustrate inflexibility. Paul, a native of Hong Kong, refused to alter his career objective when

---

[1] Story from *Guideposts,* July, 1971.

he was suddenly paralyzed in an automobile accident while he was in college. He decided, against all the odds of mounting educational and medical expenses, to continue his studies in chemical engineering at the University of Wisconsin. The adjustments he has had to make in his life-style have been staggering and certainly indicate his flexibility. He is now nearing completion of his education.

Through every step of your planning, you need to remain open and flexible. Be aware that at any stage, minor or even radical changes of plan may be called for.

Be Realistic

Imagine for a moment that a young person—let's call her Ellen—is confined to a wheelchair. She decides to become a computer operator. This is a realistic goal. There are many "wheelees" in the computer business. So Ellen takes the required training and becomes qualified for the job. Then comes the bitter test. She applies for a job at the only computer firm in her home town only to discover that the firm cannot accommodate persons in wheelchairs. Although companies are now legally obliged to make arrangements for handicapped employees, they can be forced to do so only through court action. The prospective employee in a wheelchair may face months and even years of expensive litigation before his or her rights are established. Ellen needed to get the facts about the firm she hoped to work for before she went to the time and expense of becoming qualified, assuming, of course, that she was unwilling or unable to work farther away from home.

The problem of preparing for nonexistent jobs or for jobs in over-crowded fields is not limited to handicapped persons. We heard of a young man who forged his way through years of training in agricultural research that prepared him to be of great value to foreign, developing countries. On his first overseas assignment, he discovered he really didn't like living abroad despite a high salary and fringe benefits. Since his specialty was not in demand in the U.S., he had to acquire still more training in another aspect of agricultural chemistry before he became employable.

CONCLUSION

You can for the most part only approach the future one step at a time. Usually you cannot find a job with a future until you have finished high school. You cannot find a position in your chosen career until you have completed the needed training. Move one step at a time, but plan as far ahead as possible. The way to start is by researching several career areas in which you are interested. The next chapter tells you how to go about this. Begin now to make your preliminary lists and plans. If you do, you will be positioning yourself well on the launching pad toward a successful future in the challenging and changing world of work.

CHAPTER II

Getting Started—The Research Stage

MAKING UP YOUR MIND

If you have started your career game plan, or even if you have just thought about it, you have probably discovered one thing. In order to progress very far with any plan, you have to make a lot of important decisions. We're not talking about deciding what career area you will train for. That decision will come later. We are talking about the hundreds of little and big decisions you need to make along the way. For example, do you know of one or two career areas you are enough interested in already to go to the trouble of finding out more about them? What areas do you think you would find most satisfying? Which pay the most? How important is money to you anyway? What career would you be physically and mentally best able to handle? For which do you think you could obtain needed financing for education and training? And so on and on.

"What do you want to be when you grow up?" It is a question most children have been asked many times by adults trying to make conversation. Now when they inquire about what you plan to do when you finish school they expect you to have made a lot of these decisions and to have selected a career direction. You will probably get a lot of unasked for advice. The final decisions, the ones that will shape your life-style in the future, must be made by you.

"Very few people know how to go about making a choice. While most people take a look at some of the advantages and disadvantages of making a certain decision, they attack decision-making without being clear about what is really important to them," said Gordon Porter Miller, a consultant on decision-making to corporations and educational institutions. Here are some tips that will make you a better and a faster decision-maker.

Procrastinating

Procrastination is the first enemy of decision-making. You will probably never have time to sit down and go through the whole planning process suggested in the previous chapter, but don't put off starting. You can always find time to jot down a few items on a list. The time to jot them down is when they occur to you. Make a habit of always having a pencil at hand. You can gather up the pieces of paper later to sort them and include them in your more complete plan.

Stewing Around

Don't stew around mentally. One of the authors has a cat who goes through this process every time she wants out. When you hold the door open she sniffs and looks all around. She can't seem to make up her mind. Counting to ten hurries her decision occasionally. More often than not, the door closes with her on the inside.

Stewing around can effectively block or delay your decision-making. The way to get out of the stew is to take some action. Suppose when you start to plan you wind up with a list of two dozen areas you think you want to know more about. If you can't decide, close your eyes and put your finger on the list. Begin your information search with the item on which it falls. This will allow you to keep going rather than stew around. Sooner or later, the direction will straighten itself out if the area you chose was not the best. If you do not keep moving ahead, you cannot even find this out.

Daydreaming

Daydreaming may be another stumbling block. Your dreams should play an important part in your planning. The danger is that you can get stuck in the dreaming stage. You may know a person who talks about writing a book but never really does anything about it. In his or her dreams he or she is already an acclaimed author who receives huge royalties and nationwide publicity. A wise father once told his child, "Always remember you can be anything or do anything in this world if you want it badly enough and if you are willing to work hard enough and long enough." Let your wants and dreams set the direction of your career plan, but don't forget to include necessary time for training and hard work.

Handling Frustration

Use your frustration tolerance constructively. Most handicapped people have developed a very high tolerance for frustration. It is a way of coping with the many difficult situations in which they find themselves. A high frustration tolerance level can help you to keep on your career pathway when obstacles seem to hold you back. Be sure you don't use it to support your tendency to procrastinate or stew around.

FACTORS BEYOND YOUR CONTROL

> The best laid schemes o' mice and men
> Gang aft a-gley [often go awry];
> An' lea'e us nought but grief and pain,
> For promis'd joy.

These lines written by Robert Burns in the eighteenth century have been often quoted by practical people. Careful career planning is a way to gain control over your future work life. Yet if you are a practical person, you have already realized that plans can come to naught if you have not considered the factors over which you have little or no control. The general state of the economy, how this affects changing needs in the job market, and the location of available jobs are three such factors that affect everyone, especially those coming into the job market for the first time.

The Economy

Whether we are having a recession or a boom affects all new job seekers. Recessions cause a rise in unemployment and the layoff of many employees. Union seniority rules require the last hired to be the first fired. In such times, the newly trained person seeking his first job is competing with experienced persons for a decreasing number of jobs.

Whether the country is at war or at peace also affects the economy and individuals. When an expanding military need draws off many young men, the resulting shortage of workers may create opportunities for beginners. But these men usually return. Any Vietnam veteran can tell you a personal story of the disruptions in his career plans that war caused.

The Job Market

Today's teenagers will be entering the job market just following that extraordinary population bulge known as the post-World War II baby boom. These people will still be in the work force. The Bureau of

Labor Statistics projects that in 1982 there were 110 million workers with and without jobs in the prime age group of 25 to 54 years of age. By 1995 the labor force is projected to be about 131 million—an increase of about 19 percent. Predictions are for fierce competition for promotions, some career disappointments, and the need for career goal readjustments. The population bulge has already caused changes in the plans of many who trained for teaching careers and found no jobs available. School populations are now decreasing as the bulge moves on.

The job market is strongly influenced by technological progress. As soon as television became an industry, it created the need for thousands of persons to fill new kinds of jobs. The computer industry, which is advancing more rapidly than any other at the present time, is daily creating jobs that never existed before. As it advances it also abolishes many routine jobs in the clerical, communications, and manufacturing fields. Right from the start of your planning, give careful thought to whether the field you consider is in an expanding or contracting industry.

Location

The geographic location of available jobs must be considered unless you are prepared to move anywhere in the country that jobs or careers exist. If you prefer to stay in the area where you are, or if you would like to move to the West, the Southwest, or the South, for example, you must consider what is available in the area of your choice. A now retired steel company executive admits, "I never intended to go into the steel business, but that is the kind of business there was in this town." Hundreds of miners and factory workers will tell you that they went into the mines or factories because their fathers or mothers worked there. It was the main kind of work available. Many who entered at low-level entry jobs were able to work their way up through on-the-job training and experience.

MAKING IT TO THE TOP

The above three factors have affected every young person entering the work force throughout history. Handicapped persons have to contend with limitations placed upon them by their handicaps. For some of you, these may be the overriding conditions over which you have no control. For example, a blind person cannot hope to become a graphic artist or a flight controller. A person in a wheelchair cannot become a professional baseball player or a plumber, but no matter what your handicap is, the choice is always much broader than you may imagine. Consider this list of examples just to get your thinking started.

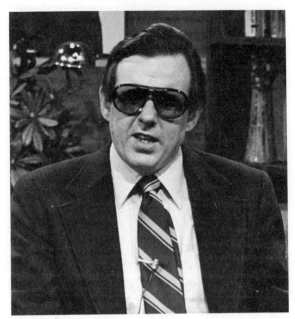

Ed Walker

Nansie S. Sharpless, PhD, is a research biochemist on the faculty of Albert Einstein College of Medicine. She lost her hearing as a result of a severe illness when she was fourteen.

Dawnelle Cruze is a social worker who was born blind. She works at the Tidewater Chapter of the American Red Cross.

Dave Harmon, who became a quadraplegic as the result of an automobile accident, is completing his internship in pharmacy at Greenville General Hospital in South Carolina.

Gene Williams, another quadraplegic accident victim, is enjoying success as a jazz musician.

Dennis Smith works as a sheet-metal worker for the General Electric Company in spite of his epilepsy.

Ed Walker is a blind-from-birth radio announcer and television co-host for a talk show on Channel 7 in Washington, D.C.

Max Cleland, head of the Veterans Administration in Washington, lost his legs and one arm in the Vietnam war.

Robert Menchel, deaf from the age of seven, is a senior physicist with the Xerox Corporation.

Henry Henscheid is Director of Advocacy and Consultant of Rights

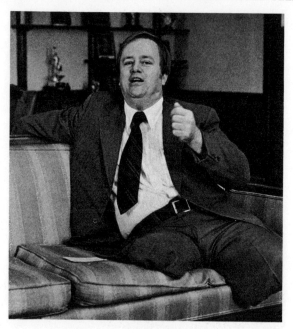

for forty-seven affiliates of the California Easter Seal Society. He was born with cerebral palsy.

Laureen Summers is a weaver, designer, and teacher of weaving in Silver Spring, Maryland, who also has cerebral palsy.

Jo Ann Haseltine of California is an administrator and founder of "The Puzzle People," an organization for learning-disabled people. She is herself learning-disabled.

Birdie Minor is a speech pathologist and supervisor of speech pathology and therapy at the Woodrow Wilson Rehabilitation Center in Virginia. She was put in a wheelchair by polio.

Bill Sayers, a respiratory polio quadraplegic who spent fifteen years in the hospital, is coauthor with his wife of a successful book. He is now at work on another and is the author of numerous articles and short stories.

Clare Jo Schnitz of El Paso, Texas, is another respiratory polio quadraplegic who earns some money and some satisfaction by tutoring college students in English.

Ann McDaniels is a blind long-distance operator for Southwestern Bell.

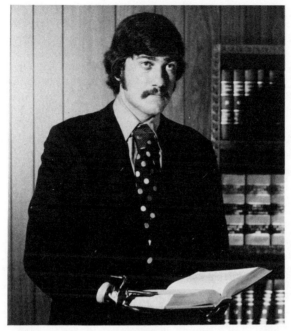

John Kemp

John Kemp heads his own law firm in Kansas although he was born without arms or legs.

Robert Sampson, who is a quadraplegic caused by muscular dystrophy contracted in childhood, is a vice-president of United Airlines.

This list could go on and on of handicapped and disabled people who have found their way to an amazing variety of successful careers. Begin your search with a completely open mind. At the beginning of your planning, don't limit your options by limiting your thinking.

FINDING HELP—CAREER GUIDANCE

Part of the problem for young people seeking to enter the labor force is the fact that there are so many kinds of work. No one person making his or her choice can possibly know about more than a handful of these. Among the ones you don't know about may be the one that is just right for you. This is where a career guidance counselor or a rehabilitation counselor can be of special help. A professional counselor can help you:

- to broaden your knowledge of many kinds of work and careers;
- to discover more specifically your aptitudes, interests, and talents through a battery of aptitude, achievement, and interest tests;
- to find general information about a number of career areas for which you show aptitude and in which you are interested;
- to find out what special education or training you need for your chosen field;
- to locate scholarships or other financial aids for needed education or training; and
- to guide as you apply for and obtain your first job in your chosen field.

The support of a guidance or rehabilitation counselor can be helpful at every stage of your preparation for your adult work life, from making the decisions on what areas to look into to assisting you with obtaining your first job. Counselors also help older people who need to change their lines of work or to reassess their talents and skills.

We have used the terms rehabilitation counselor and vocational guidance counselor interchangeably up to now. Actually they are not the same, and both may offer services of use to you in your search for a meaningful career. Vocational guidance counselors are of service to all kinds of people whether handicapped or not. They may have a broader range of information about types of work. They usually do not have special training for, or skill in handling, job-related or training-related special problems sometimes encountered by handicapped persons. Rehabilitation counselors are trained to assist handicapped persons with their special problems in all areas of life. They are usually well acquainted with the kinds of work handicapped persons can do and with ways of becoming employed if you are handicapped.

The kind of counselor to serve you best will depend on your special needs but particularly on what kind of counselor is available to you in the area in which you live.

WHERE THE JOBS WILL BE IN THE 1990's

Every good career plan is two-sided. One side faces you and reflects accurately your abilities, needs, potential talents, dreams, and desires. The other side faces the society in which you live and reflects the skills, talents, abilities, and services it needs. You and your guidance counselor can work out a plan that weaves a web between these two sides.

Reports by the U.S. Labor Department predict the ten fastest-growing occupational areas—ones where the number of jobs is expected to rise 40 percent or more by 1995. The career areas and minimum expected change in total employment are:

Computer systems analysts	217,000
Computer programmers	205,000
Computer operators	160,000
Electrical engineers	209,000
Electrical and electronic technicians	222,000
Nurses, registered	642,000
Receptionists	189,000
Cashiers	744,000
Guards and doorkeepers	300,000
Cooks, restaurants	149,000

Another twenty-five areas where job growth is expected to be large by 1995 and the minimum expected change in total employment are:

Accountants and auditors	344,000
Automotive mechanics	324,000
Teachers, kindergarten and elementary	511,000
Licensed practical nurses	220,000
Food preparation and service workers, fast-food restaurants	297,000
Kitchen helpers	305,000
Nursing aides and orderlies	423,000
Clerical supervisors	162,000
Lawyers	159,000
Physicians	163,000
Waiters and waitresses	562,000
Cooks, short-order, specialty, and fast food	141,000
Helpers, trades	190,000
Electrician	173,000
Bank tellers	142,000
Managers, store	292,000
General clerks, office	696,000
Secretaries	791,000
Sales representatives, technical	386,000
Carpenters	247,000
Maintenance repairers, general utility	193,000
Building custodians	779,000
Sales representatives, nontechnical	160,000
Supervisors of blue-collar workers	319,000
Salesclerks	685,000
Delivery and route workers	153,000

Statistics and reports are useful things, particularly in the early stages of your planning. They do not mean that if you have a deep interest and aptitude in one of the more crowded areas you have to give up those plans. They do mean that it may be wise to take a double major. You can prepare yourself in a second area in case you are unable to find a position in the field of your first choice.

JOBS AND EDUCATION

All the industries mentioned above will be expanding during the next few years. They will be hiring people of every educational level from high school dropouts to PhD's. We live in such a complex technological society that there will be a greater need for persons with training in every type of skill and for those with advanced education in many different fields. The need for high school dropouts continues to diminish. As a general rule, persons with more education start out with jobs that pay better. They earn more rapid promotions. Some personality factors important to on-the-job success may be shared by persons regardless of their educational achievement levels. For example, how hard you work, how quickly you learn, and how personally responsible you are all make a difference in how successful you are.

Let's take a look at what kinds of jobs are generally available for persons with differing educational backgrounds. As you read, keep in mind the career you are planning. Where do you want to fit into the picture?

High School Graduates

What is available for high school graduates who do not go on to post-high school education? Vocational high school graduates are often prepared for entry positions in the vocations for which they trained. Sometimes they may need to get further on-the-job training or join an apprenticeship program. Some high school vocational courses also offer work experience that allows a student to get a taste of the work before he or she commits more time to it.

Business graduates are also often prepared for entry-level positions in business. How good a job you can get depends on the degree of your proficiency and on your success at finding the "right" job. You may start out as a mail clerk, receptionist, typist, or file clerk, or you may start with a job requiring more skill and more responsibility as a secretary.

Courses in distributive education may also prepare you for entry-level positions in the retail trade such as salesperson, stock clerk, inventory clerk, cashier-checker, or order clerk. Both business and distributive education courses can lead to a variety of occupations in the service industries such as cleaning, food, or health service.

High school graduates as well as high school dropouts can join the competition for an ever dwindling number of jobs in unskilled labor. These include everything from general labor in the construction field, to janitorial and custodial work, to ushering in a theater or waiting on tables. There is nothing demeaning about any kind of work. All workers make some contribution to keeping our society going. The main disadvantage of such jobs is that they usually pay little and offer few opportunities for advancement.

Starting at the bottom is a well-honored American tradition. The man who formerly owned and operated the public transportation system for the District of Columbia started his business career as a junkman. American history is full of successful and famous people who started out just as humbly. The important factors in working your way up are your ability and your appetite for hard work. Many companies, when they recognize people with ability and ambition, will train them on the job or send them to special schools.

High School Graduates With Some Post-High School Training

Even a small amount of education beyond high school opens the door to many more job and career opportunities. Special training ranging from a few weeks to two or three years is available in numerous business schools, technical schools, art schools, and community colleges. Some of the courses offered lead to certification in fields where this is necessary, such as nursing or medical technology. Others, just as career-oriented, train in fields as varied as flying, cooking, and commercial art.

Some industries in need of an increasing number of trained technicians are the computer industry, the truck transportation industry, the building maintenance industry, and the health care industry.

College Graduates—Liberal Arts

The purpose for which liberal arts education was designed, some hundreds of years ago, was not to provide vocational training. Its purpose was to improve and deepen the student's understanding of our history and culture. Its primary thrust was to prepare him or her to function better as a responsible adult member of society.

Some interesting studies have been done over the years showing that college graduates as a group make more money on a monthly basis and over their lifetimes than nongraduates. This scarcely proves the economic value of a liberal arts education, since the studies included all college graduates. Most graduates, these days, take at least two of their four years of college in some sort of career-oriented or major-interest–oriented training.

What is available for the liberal arts graduate is not much different from what is available to high school graduates. It is not uncommon for applicants for positions of typist, secretary, or file clerk to be asked whether they have college degrees. It is not necessary to have a degree to do such jobs skillfully. When the competition for jobs is great, employers use such information to help them estimate the level of intelligence or competence of prospective employees. They may favor those with more education.

Not infrequently, liberal arts graduates take additional technical or business training in order to acquire a marketable skill and become employed.

College Graduates With Some Specialization

College graduates who take engineering, business practices, or any other career-oriented major usually start out a little higher and rise more quickly from their entry-level jobs.

Most four-year colleges require that a certain percentage of your studies during the first year or two be made up of liberal arts subjects. You can concentrate more on the field of your major interest during the last two years. Many students who graduate from such colleges intend to continue study in their area of major interest by attending graduate school.

Graduate Degrees

Advanced degrees earned through years of special training are necessary for the professions such as medicine and law. Advanced training is increasingly necessary in every area of science and industry. This is particularly true if you wish to move up the ladder toward the top positions.

Many persons who like to study and are good at it go ahead and earn a PhD degree. This is done with the thought of college teaching in the area of their expertise. Here is a word of caution if you think this is the way you would like to go. Be sure to look into the question of whether there will be a need for teachers of your specialty by the time you achieve your degree. College populations are declining. Be sure you are not merely delaying the moment of decision when you must go out and earn your own living. If you are a good student, you have learned how to be successful as a student. You may on a subconscious level want to cling to the pattern of success that you have established.

CONCLUSION

It is easy to get so carried away with the process of selecting a career and the many ideas that must be considered that you lose track of the most important factor of all. What would you like most to do? What would make you the happiest?

As you read about careers and talk to persons who are in them, you will discover there are some that interest and challenge you. There are others that interest you principally because they pay so well. Some lucky people are interested from the start in high-paying careers that also challenge and fascinate them. Many more have to make a decision along the way as to the relative importance of making money and doing something interesting.

Fred Mancuso, a successful Canadian artist who has spent most of the past ten years in a wheelchair, has lived through this dilemma. We would like to share some of his conclusions with you.

Fred received a minimum of art education through his brother, who paid for his first course. Although it seemed to be his natural inclination, Fred's parents were opposed to his becoming an artist. He yielded to the pressure and studied drafting, a trade that his parents felt would better prepare him to make a living.

At the age of sixteen he went to work as a mail boy. He worked his way up to senior mechanical draftsman with the same company. In his own words, "I took drafting for a living and hated it for eighteen years! No matter how small the wages may be, the one advice I can give is as long as you are happy doing whatever you are doing—this is the secret to being successful. To your self first be true. I wasn't, and I ask myself what was triggered in me to bring me to an abrupt stop in my drafting career?"

What started Fred on his new and successful career as an artist was his wife. She encouraged his interest in art and built his confidence. Now he is a full-time artist with his own studio. His paintings have won a number of prizes. He has exhibited and sold in the U.S., Canada, Europe, and Japan.

For him the most important gain is that he is happy. "Why, even after suffering the effects of multiple sclerosis, I am still the happiest person—even after hypertension, diabetes, cataracts operations, I feel like I am on top of the world." Fred stresses that "Working just because the money is good or doing a job you don't really like is a very sad thing to do. The rule is—get into a job you enjoy, no matter how small. Being at peace with yourself as I have found is worth more than all the gold in the world."

CAREER SELECTION CHECKLIST

If your career game plan is on schedule, by now you should have done most of the things summarized on the following checklist.

1. Think seriously about the career in which you would be capable and happy.
2. Talk over career possibilities with family members, counselors, teachers, friends, and persons they recommend.

3. Find a guidance or a rehabilitation counselor and discuss your career future with him or her.
4. Take any aptitude, achievement, vocational assessment, personality, and interest inventory tests your counselor recommends.
5. Study career information provided by your counselor or obtained on your own.
6. Make one or more trips to a library to study career information.
7. Send away for additional career information if needed to:

> trade or professional associations or unions;
> health and rehabilitation service agencies to gain facts and specific career information as they relate to your specific handicap.

8. Consider your proposed career in relation to where the jobs will be in the 1990's.
9. Consider your proposed career area in relationship to any physical, psychological, or mental limitations your handicap imposes.
10. Consider your proposed career choice in relation to:

> your aptitudes, interests, skills, and potential abilities;
> your future economic needs;
> your future happiness and enjoyment of life; and
> your desire to contribute—to pull your own weight in society to the fullest extent possible.

11. Check through the resources section following this list to discover if you need to send for information. Make another visit to the library. Write to appropriate organizations before you can complete this career selection phase of your game plan.

SELECTED RESOURCES CHAPTER II— CAREER SELECTION

Notes: Information has been listed in this section in the order the subjects were discussed earlier in the chapter.

Some listed publications are free, some cost a little, and some are expensive. Ask the price, or include a line saying "Send only if it costs less than $1.00 or $5.00" or whatever.

* indicates books that can usually be found in public libraries or in your guidance or rehabilitation counselor's office.

SELF-ANALYSIS

The Career Emphasis series consists of six skills-oriented workbooks based on accepted models of career development. It is designed specifically to meet needs of adults ages eighteen and over who are facing the added responsibilities that accompany adulthood. *Emphasis: Decisions; Emphasis: Self; Emphasis: Work; Emphasis: Preparation; Emphasis: Change.* Olympus Publishing Co., 1670 East Thirteenth South, Salt Lake City, UT 84105.

Miller, Gordon Porter. *Life Choices: How to Make the Critical Decisions—About Your Education, Career, Marriage, Family.* Thomas Y. Crowell.

FINDING CAREER COUNSELING SERVICES

Career Guidance Counselors

If you attend a public or private school, see what guidance services are available. If none, perhaps the school can recommend an approved guidance service center.

Call your county's school system headquarters, which is usually in the county seat. Ask to speak to the person supervising guidance and counseling. He or she may be able to put you in touch with a guidance counselor nearby. Public schools are now legally required to make such services available to the handicapped who meet age or other general requirements.

Write to the National Rehabilitation Association, 633 South Washington Street, Alexandria, VA 22314. Ask for the *Journal of Rehabilitation* and the newsletter.

Write to *B'nai B'rith Career and Counseling Services*, 1640 Rhode Island Avenue, NW, Washington, DC 20036. This national office issues more than 80 publications, including a quarterly magazine. Ask for the location of the nearest B'nai B'rith office that offers guidance and testing services. You may find an office listed in your local phone book.

Write to or call the voluntary health agency that serves people with your particular disability. Some have counseling services. Talk to the social worker or the intake worker. He or she may have some suggestions as to where you can find the services you need. (There is a list of headquarters offices for selected national health agencies in the Appendix if you are unable to find a local office in the phone book.)

Rehabilitation Counselors

Rehabilitation counselors are employed by the federal and state governments. They can be found through regional and state offices. There is a list in the Appendix.

GATHERING CAREER INFORMATION

For the Handicapped

For information on special programs in art for the handicapped, write to National Arts and the Handicapped Information Service, Arts and Special Constituencies Project, National Endowment for the Arts, 2401 E Street, NW, Room 1200, Washington, DC 20506.

For information on special opportunities in the sciences for the handicapped, write to Project on the Handicapped in Science, Office of Opportunities in Science, American Association for the Advancement of Science, 1776 Massachusetts Avenue, NW, Washington, DC 20036.

Write to Closer Look, P.O. Box 1492, Washington, DC 20013. Ask for the bibliographies.

Write to President's Committee on Employment of the Handicapped, 1111 20th Street, NW, Washington, DC 20210. Ask for free career information publications.

For the Nonhandicapped

One of the responsibilities of your guidance counselor or rehabilitation counselor is to help you find information about careers. If you want to begin a search on your own, the following are good starting points for finding career information written for the general, nonhandicapped reader.

Make a trip to the library. Spend a day or more studying the latest edition of the U.S. Department of Labor's *Occupational Outlook Handbook*. This 363-page encyclopedia of careers covers several hundred occupations in major industries. For each it covers: what the work is like, job prospects, personal qualifications, education and training, earnings, chances for advancement, and where to find additional information.

Note: The above book should be ordered from the U.S. Department of Labor, Bureau of Labor Statistics, U.S. Government Printing Office, Washington, DC, 20402, for $8.50 in paperback. Make checks payable to the Superintendent of Documents.

The Guide for Occupational Exploration. U.S. Department of Labor, Employment and Training Administration, 1979. Groups occupations by interests and by ability and traits required for successful performance. *Dictionary of Occupational Titles.* U.S. Department of Labor, Employment and Training Administration, U.S. Employment Service.

Write to the trade or professional association that represents the business or profession in which you are interested. Ask them to send any career information. They may include information on training programs and on scholarships, fellowships, and loans. They may also have some special programs to assist the handicapped.

Note: In order to find the address of the association in your interest area, call the information service of your public library. They usually will look it up for you, often on the same call. If it takes longer, they will call you back.

PUBLICATIONS YOU CAN SEND FOR

For starters, write to the Federal Government Jobs, Office of Personnel Management, Washington, DC 20415. Ask for BRE-78 or *U.S. Government Organizations with Positions Outside the Competitive Civil Service.* Also, ask for BRE-8 or *Employment of Physically Handicapped Persons in the Federal Service,* and any other materials they may have relating to your area of interest.

For information on Civil Service careers, write to the U.S. Department of State, Recruitment Division, P.O. Box 12209, Rosslyn Station, Arlington, VA 22209.

Mainstream is a publication that lists all aspects of employment for the handicapped and can be a useful guide. Write to *Mainstream,* 1200 15th Street, NW, Washington, DC 20005.

Area Trends: In Employment and Unemployment, U.S. Department of Labor, Employment and Training Administration, Washington, DC 20213, lists labor surplus areas by state. This statistical booklet can help you identify areas of employment availability in your state.

The Bureau of Labor Statistics publishes a quarterly bulletin that occasionally focuses on specific careers such as English, Ecology, Clerical Work, Foreign Languages, Health, Liberal Arts, Math, Mechanics, Outdoors, Science, and Social Studies. The articles discuss the types of jobs that may be available to persons with an interest in or proficiency in a particular academic field.

CHAPTER III

Finding the Right School

How much do you like going to school? Do you get satisfaction out of learning things, studying, reading and writing? Or would you rather do almost anything else? Those who get the most out of their post-high school education are usually those who study the hardest. Of course, it is always more fun when you are learning something that really turns you on and mastering skills you need to get started on your career.

Many handicapped people feel that they want to get all the education they can. They feel it will compensate in some small way for their disability. The following thoughts, some of them in the handicapped person's own words, indicate how important they feel education was to them.

Birdie Minor, speech pathologist whom you met in Chapter II, says, "My education is extremely important to me, since I am a speech pathologist, which required a master's degree. If I didn't have my education, I don't know what I'd be doing today— certainly something not as satisfactory as what I'm doing now."

Henry Hooton of Eugene, Oregon, is an intellectually disabled custodian who stresses the importance of getting your vocational rehabilitation counselor to find education and training offered by private organizations, community colleges, and on-the-job training programs. Continuing education courses are often available that emphasize personal and social development and the development of job skills and special interests.

Thomas Lyczko of Amsterdam, New York, is a hearing- and vision-handicapped college student. "I think you should go to the best college you can get into, because that's where you will be challenged the most and hopefully learn the most."

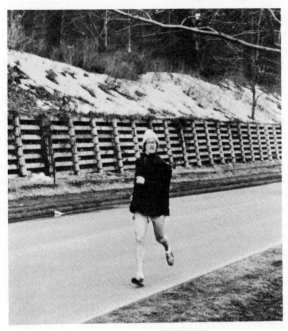

*Thomas Lyczko nears the finish of the Club Marathon at Suny/
Albany in 1977. He set a personal record of 3:22, which he lowered
to 3:12 in 1979.*

With the help of his future wife, who typed his papers, writer *Bill
Sayers* took a correspondence course in short-story writing while he
was still in the hospital in an iron lung.

Jo Ann Haseltine, learning-disabled federal employee, says, "Sensory
integration training does not always work for every child or adult,
but for me it was the number one therapy in making my life become
a success rather than a continuous series of failures."

Andrew Stamm of Seattle, Washington, who is now well into a career
in art, was originally diagnosed as a child with autism and severe language disability. Speaking of his art training, Andrew's mother says:
"What has art been for Andrew? It originally helped his teachers and
family to open the doors of his mind. Now he can read, write, compose
letters, and do mathematics. Art has given him self-confidence. It's
been his means of acceptance into the 'normal' world—his means of
expression."

Laurine Summers is a cerebral palsied artist who lives and works
in Takoma Park, Maryland. She is a designer and teacher of weaving.

She is adamant about education. "Find a place suited to your needs. Demand the best education that is good for you. I found a small school that paid a lot of attention to the individual, a place where I could design my own course of study."

TYPES OF SCHOOLS

In the process of selecting your career area or areas, you have probably already learned a good deal about how much additional training or education you need. The following information will help you by limiting the selection of schools to those that offer what you need. It is a good thing, because there are more than 3,000 colleges and universities in the United States. There are more than 8,500 special post-secondary schools, including business schools, technical schools, computer schools, flight schools, cosmetology/barber schools, art schools, music conservatories, and many more.

Often special training schools, junior colleges, and colleges may offer training for the same career area. The choice is a wide one. One of the first steps is to decide on a general type of school. Before you tackle that decision, define as specifically as you can what kind of school you need. Here is a rundown of the general types of school.

Four-year Colleges and Universities

The general university is made up of one or more undergraduate colleges as well as graduate professional schools and colleges. It typically has a large enrollment. Usually it has a greater variety of courses and major fields of study than do other types of post-secondary institutions. It usually provides a more extensive library and better physical education, laboratory, and recreational facilities than do smaller schools. It may offer preprofessional training at the undergraduate level and professional training through its graduate schools.

Smaller Four-year Colleges

The typical liberal arts college enrollment is much smaller than at a general university—ranging from 200 to 2,500+ students. These schools generally emphasize liberal arts as a background preparation for later professional training at a university or professional school.

Schools Offering Four-year Programs in Special Fields

Engineering, technology, and physical sciences are offered in four-year programs at a small number of specialized technical schools. Similarly a small number of schools specialize in programs in the fine arts. These schools usually offer a limited number of liberal arts subjects. They concentrate on technical courses that lead to the growth and development of skills necessary for their graduates to enter their chosen fields of work.

State-supported Schools

A good education at below average cost can be had at tax-supported state colleges. Teachers' colleges in many states now offer programs in liberal arts and are changing over to state college status. State colleges and universities may offer broader programs and include professional training in various graduate schools.

Two-year Community and Private Colleges

There are now over 1,000 community colleges supported by a combination of state and local funds. There are over 300 private two-year colleges. These schools provide the first two years of college-level training for students who plan to go on to earn a degree at another college or university. They also provide vocational-technical training for students who will be terminating their higher education. Tuition at publicly supported community colleges is usually either low or free to residents of the area. It is not uncommon for these schools to accept all students who have diplomas from accredited local high schools in the community. Students with mediocre high school records are not as likely to be accepted in many four-year institutions. They may use the two-year college as a stepping-stone to raise their readiness for college-level work. If you are thinking of going this route, check out the school from which you plan to graduate to be sure all your credits will be accepted. (For a directory of transfer information see the resources section.)

Schools with Special Programs of Usually Less than Two Years

In almost every city you will find a wide variety of special schools offering programs ranging from a few weeks to a few years. These include many vocational schools, beauty/barber schools, business schools, schools of commercial art or photography, and many more.

Many skilled trades are learned through apprenticeship or on-the-job training. This training may last for several years while the apprentice is paid increasing amounts as he or she progresses. A booklet on apprenticeships is listed in the resources section.

Nontraditional Post-secondary Education

In recent years some colleges and universities have developed external degree programs. These offer college course credit for nonclassroom learning experiences such as correspondence work, radio or TV courses, independent study, travel, work and volunteer experience, and passing written examinations. These programs, first developed to accommodate students who hold full-time jobs, are often particularly useful to handicapped students.

The University of Oklahoma offers an external degree program in which students are not usually present for any extended period on the campus. The State University of New York, the Community College of Vermont, and many others offer similar programs.

One can also get much of one's education through correspondence courses. The Correspondence Study Division of the National University Extension Association can help you locate ones you need. You will find their address in the resources section.

Degree-directed students should check with the college from which they wish to graduate as to whether the college will accept correspondence credits.

Some members of the National University Extension Association require only that 25 percent of the degree requirement be campus-based.

The National Home Study Council, 1601 18th Street, NW, Washington, DC 20009, issues a free catalogue listing hundreds of correspondence courses at the high schools and college levels.

If you are not interested in earning college credit, you may want to investigate some of the more than 100 free universities, which offer a wide variety of courses. They often have no admission requirements and low tuition fees. They may be associated with large universities. Generally they offer courses in areas not covered by traditional academic courses. For a source list, see resources section.

NARROWING YOUR CHOICE

The Public Library—A Good Place to Start

The best way to find out about an individual school or university is to study its catalog put out every year. Such catalogs, often very large, describe the various courses offered, including the required courses for various majors. They also give tuition and fee costs and rates for food and lodging. They define student personnel services, extracurricular activities available, and much more. Colleges have recently begun to charge for copies of their catalogs. In the interest of saving space on your bookshelf, as well as a little money, you may want to go to the library. Most public libraries have collections of college catalogs, as well as many college directories and directories of other schools. A librarian can help you narrow your choice to six or eight, and then you can write for your own copies of those catalogs. Read catalogs critically. They stress the assets, not the limitations of a school. In these early stages of your search, be sure you consider the following:

Quality Education and Location Factors. In general the Ivy League and Big Ten schools offer high-quality education, but so do many little-known colleges. A degree from one of the latter, however, does not offer the status of a degree from an Ivy League school or a Big Ten university. At the other end of the spectrum, one must be wary of so-called diploma mills that offer college degrees by mail. One good way of establishing the minimum quality standards of a school you are considering is to look it up in the Council on Post-Secondary Accreditation directory. The COPA publishes a directory annually. It is listed in the resource section.

Schools specialize in different areas. Usually the best schools for training in one career area are listed in the career literature about that area. For example, if you already know that you want to specialize in nuclear engineering, or hotel management, you may have to investigate only a handful of schools. The same is true of the technical institutes and vocational schools. If you want a quality education in a highly specialized area, the location of the best schools will be the determining factor.

Sometimes there are nonacademic geographical considerations. Perhaps for financial reasons, you need to get at least part of your education while living at home and commuting to college. Perhaps you are looking for a school in a certain city where you have a friend or relative who would rent you a room and provide board. Perhaps you are in a wheelchair; your choice will be influenced by whether the school has accessible buildings. To check on these considerations, refer to the end of this chapter and the chapter entitled "Your Legal Rights as a Handicapped Person." Remember that narrowing your options is an important part of the process to decision-making.

Check the Admissions Policy. Remarkable strides have been made in accommodating handicapped students at all kinds of schools since the legislation of 1973. Not all schools have made all adjustments. You must check out every school under consideration to determine if it meets particular needs posed by your handicap. Some books that help with this checking are listed in the resources section.

Meeting Admission Standards. In addition to your high school records, most colleges make use of the Scholastic Aptitude Test or SAT scores. These tests are administered six times a year by the College Entrance Examination Board. In most high schools they are given during the junior year and again in the senior year.

A second widely used testing program is the American College Testing program, or ACT. It is given five times a year during the junior and senior years.

The tests attempt to measure your educational achievement in a number of areas and the level of skills like reading, writing, and mathematics that are necessary to pursue further education. They also measure readiness and maturity factors needed to succeed in college. These are aptitude tests. It is not intended that a student be able to study for them. The best preparation is constant and well-organized habits of work throughout your school career, as well as a good night's sleep before the test.

How Much Will It Cost? It is, of course, quite impossible for most people to consider attending a college or school without determining how much it will cost and finding ways and means of meeting the expenses. Most schools have scholarships, awards, and loan funds for which you may be eligible. Admissions officers are helpful in checking all possibilities and helping you find ways to finance your education. There are also federal and state funds available to help handicapped people finance education. Your rehabilitation counselor can help you locate these funds. Banks offer educational loan programs. Insurance policies may cover some of the costs. Most parents try to set aside some money for their children's education.

To finance the years of education most students and their families put together a patchwork of sums of money from a wide variety of sources such as those mentioned above. In fact, there are so many possibilities that the subject of financing your post-high school education is covered in more detail in the next chapter.

When to Send for Catalogs. The time has come for you to obtain your own copies of school catalogs. You have now boiled down your list of possible schools to five or six. Send for catalogs for each of these so that you can study them in detail. Read them critically to get an accurate picture. At the same time you can ask for any printed information on scholarships and loans. Many schools have free pamphlets or catalogs listing student aid and loan programs. Prepare a tally sheet for each school. Then prepare a numbered list of questions for which you need answers, for each of the schools. Each person's list of questions will be different, of course. We suggest the following starter list:

1. Does the school offer a fully accredited, quality course of study in the area of my interest?

2. Will the school help me find needed financial aid? Does it have a scholarship, fellowship, or loan program?

3. Will my test scores and high school records qualify me for entrance? (Your estimate.)

4. Are the school's administrative and classroom buildings and dormitories architecturally accessible to me?

5. Is the school willing to make any special arrangements needed to accommodate the needs of a handicapped person like myself? Are there acceptable substitutes for required courses that I may not be able to take? (Examples: physical education and some laboratory courses.)

6. List additional questions that apply to you specifically.

As you study the catalogs, note down the answers to these questions on a tally sheet for each school. When you have finished, it will be a lot easier to compare the sheets than to dig through the various catalogs. There will probably be some questions for which the catalogs furnish insufficient information. Mark these with a check mark. You can then write to the college for additional facts. Before you write, be sure you read the next chapter, because you are likely to find some questions related to financial aid that need to go into the letter.

Visiting Colleges. Before making a final choice, you will want to visit any schools you are seriously considering. Check out all the facilities—classrooms, libraries, laboratories, student personnel offices, dining halls, dormitories, and facilities for extracurricular activities. Check the architectural accessibility of buildings or dormitories you will need to enter.

Write ahead to arrange for appointments with the admissions officer or any others he suggests to check out possible adaptations to your special needs. Talk to the registrar, professors, instructors, and students. Get the feel of the place. A visit also gives you a chance to see the town, if any, in which the college is located. It is important to consider your personal reaction to any place in which you are planning to spend several years of your life.

One relatively inexpensive way to visit colleges is with a college caravan. The college caravan is an organized, guided inspection tour of several colleges by a group of interested high school students. Typically, the caravan charters a bus, obtains group rates from motels or hotels, and includes on the tour a trained counselor and several chaperones. In this way expenses are reduced, but all the schools you want to see may not be included. You and some interested fellow students might talk to the school's guidance counselor about arranging a caravan. If you are a member or a client of one of the organizations serving the handicapped, someone there may be able to help you organize a smaller caravan for a group of handicapped students. Check with one of the counselors in the guidance office of your school or with the vocational rehabilitation organization in your city.

TENTATIVE CONCLUSION

The new legislation on behalf of the handicapped has greatly expanded your opportunities to get the kind of education you want. This increase in possibilities has made the selection more difficult and more time-consuming. When you do find the right school it will be worth every bit of the effort that goes into finding it. *Birdie Minor,* whom you heard from earlier in this chapter, has this to say about going to college:

"When I began looking for a college in my senior year of high school, I found it very difficult to find one that would accommodate me; therefore, I settled for a major in secretarial science. After two years of business classes, I realized that I was barking up the wrong tree and dropped out. I then began looking for a school in other states that offered a major in speech pathology. I almost went to the University of Southern Illinois, which was one of the few schools adapted for wheelchairs.

"At the same time my brother was also planning to enter college. He offered to go with me to college if I went to Florida. We both applied at several Florida schools, and we wound up going to Florida State University. It was not adapted for wheelchairs, but between my brother and friends I had very few problems getting around on campus. I thoroughly enjoyed it.

"I went to the University of Missouri for graduate study. I went there mainly because it was modified for the handicapped. It was a good experience being with other handicapped persons there. We had rap sessions that aired our many concerns and problems. It was a real growing experience for me."

SCHOOL SELECTION CHECKLIST

By the end of this chapter, if your game plan is on schedule, you should have:

1. Taken or arranged to take the SAT or ACT college entrance examinations.
2. Investigated a number of schools and types of schools in a library, and discussed them with your guidance or rehabilitation counselor and your parents.
3. Selected the best-suited type of school (e.g., two-year college, four-year college, business school, art institute).
4. Boiled down your selection to five or six that seemed most possible and written to them to obtain:

catalogs;

admissions applications;

information about financial aid programs and free booklets on financial aid; and

appointments to visit the most promising schools.

5. Visited as many as possible of the schools you are considering to:

talk to admissions officer or registrar;

talk to the financial aid officer;

talk to students, professors, townspeople, graduates; and

make your own estimate of how well you might function at that school and how well the school would meet your special needs as a handicapped person.

6. Begun filling out applications for admission to the three or four schools you would be pleased to attend if you were admitted and could work out the financing.

   Note: Since applications for admission and for financial aid are usually considered together, you will need to read the following chapter before actually sending off the applications.

7. Checked through the resources section following this list to discover if you need to send for anything, make another visit to the library, or write more letters before you can complete this selection stage.

SELECTED RESOURCES CHAPTER III— FINDING THE RIGHT SCHOOL

Notes: Information has been listed in this section in the order the subjects were discussed earlier in the chapter.

Some listed publications are free, some cost a little, and some are expensive. Ask the price, or include a line saying "Send only if it costs less than $1.00 or $5.00" or whatever.

*indicates books that can usually be found in public libraries or in your guidance or rehabilitation counselor's office.

DIFFERENT TYPES OF SCHOOLS

For information on *undergraduate colleges* consult *The College Handbook* published by the College Entrance Examination Board.

Barron's Handbook of Colleges and Universities. Barron's Educational Service, 113 Crossways Park Drive, Woodbury, NY 11797.

National Association of Trade and Technical Schools, 2021 L Street, NW, Washington, DC 20036. Ask for the list of trade and technical schools that provide accreditation.

For information on two-year and junior colleges, write to American Association of Community and Junior Colleges, 1 Dupont Circle, NW, Washington, DC 20036.

Apprenticeship Programs, a book by William Shanahan (Arco, 1983) provides information on apprenticeship programs.

*Barron's Handbook of College Transfer Information. Barron's Educational Service, Woodbury, New York.

NONTRADITIONAL TYPES OF EDUCATION

General

Credit For What You Know. An educational fact sheet containing details of how to obtain college credit without formal teaching. Published by Consumer Information, Pueblo, CO 81009.

A Guide to Educational Programs in Noncollegiate Organizations, The American Council on Education, Office of Education Credit, 1 Dupont Circle, NW Washington, DC 20036. They will evaluate courses that you have already taken to determine whether you may receive college credit for them.

Correspondence

Peterson's NOCEA Guide to Independent Study Through Correspondence Instruction, Peterson's Guides, Book Order Department, P.O. Box 978, Edison, NJ 08817.

For information on correspondence study write to the Correspondence Study Division of the National University Extension Association, Suite 360, 1 Dupont Circle, NW, Washington, DC 20036.

Homebound Study

Home Study Opportunities, a free pamphlet published by B'nai B'rith Career and Counseling Service, 1640 Rhode Island Avenue, NW, Washington, DC 20036.

Careers for the Homebound—Home Study Educational Opportunities, a pamphlet published by the President's Committee on Employment of the Handicapped, Washington, DC 20402.

For information on accredited home study programs write to the National Home Study Council, 1601 18th Street, NW, Washington, DC 20009.

External Degree Programs

On Campus–Off Campus Degree Programs for Part-Time Students, published by the National Extension Association, Suite 360, 1 Dupont Circle, NW, Washington, DC 20036.

For information on *external degree programs* write to External Degree Program Chairman, East Central College Consortium, c/o Hiram College, Hiram, OH 44234.

Accreditation

*Accredited Institutions of Post-Secondary Education. The so-called COPA directory may be purchased annually from the Publications Division of the American Council on Education, Suite 826, 1 Dupont Circle, NW, Washington, DC 20036.

SPECIAL HELP FOR THE HANDICAPPED

Getting Through College with a Disability. A summary of services available on 500 campuses for students with handicapping conditions; published by President's Committee on Employment of the Handicapped, Washington, DC 20210.

* The College Guide for Students with Disabilities. A detailed directory of higher education services, programs, and facilities accessible to handicapped students in the United States. By Elinor Gollay and Alwina Bennett. ABT Publications, 55 Wheeler Street, Cambridge, MA 02138.

Address List of Regional and Sub-Regional Libraries for the Blind and Physically Handicapped. The Library of Congress, Division for the Blind and Physically Handicapped, Washington, DC 20542.

Appleby, Judith. *Training Programs and Placement Services—Vocational Training and Placement of the Severely Handicapped.* Olympus Publishing Co., Salt Lake City, Utah. Designed for professional use, this helpful book may be found in the library or at your counselor's office.

A Chance to Go to College: A Directory of 800 Colleges that Have Special Help for Students from Minorities and Low Income Families, published by the College Entrance Examination Board, 888 7th Avenue, New York, NY 10019.

A Guide to College/Career Programs for Deaf Students, Office of Demographic Studies, Gallaudet College, Kendall Green, Washington, DC 20002. Ask for the reference booklet.

National Directory of Four-year Colleges, Two-year Colleges and Post-High School Training Programs for Young People with Learning Disabilities, Partners in Publishing, P.O. Box 50347, Tulsa, Oklahoma 74150.

COLLEGE ADMISSION TESTS

First ask your guidance counselor or high school principal about tests offered in your school.

For additional information write directly to:

College Entrance Examination Board, 888 Seventh Avenue, New York, NY 10019.

American College Testing Program, P.O. Box 168, Iowa City, IA 52240.

CHAPTER IV

Financing Your Education

There is probably no other country in the world where a prospective student has such a wide choice of ways to finance his or her higher education. "It's utter chaos!" said a young refugee from Vietnam. "In my country, the government pays for your education all the way through college." It may seem comforting to think that it would be better to have the government pay for all our educational needs throughout life. But one must remember, where there is only one source of funding, there is usually only one source of decision-making. The educational authority decides who will and who will not go on to college. It often selects those occupations which, in its judgment, the country most needs. That decision stands! It determines the whole future course of the young person's life.

In this country it is hard to imagine that a young person who is determined to get a higher education could ever run out of possible sources of funding to check out. Indeed, hundreds of sources are mentioned in this book, and that is far from all there are.

It can be chaotic, as the Vietnamese girl said, but when you get right down to it, there are only three ways you can pay for your education: (1) you can locate scholarships, fellowships, awards, or grants; (2) you can borrow through special college or other educational loan funds; and (3) you can pay outright from family resources or your own savings and earnings from summer jobs and part-time school-year jobs. It is possible to use any one of these methods. Most students use a combination of all three.

ESTIMATING YOUR EXPENSES

As you study the catalogs of the schools in which you are most interested, you will probably realize that you are going to need several thousand dollars a year to cover expenses. It is never too soon to start locating ways and means of financing your education. The financial situation can greatly influence your final choice of college.

In the last chapter you prepared a tally sheet of pertinent facts about each of five or six possible schools. This will help you to organize the whole process of locating funds. Now add a second page, a financial tally sheet, to each school's report. Go through the catalogs again. Fill in pertinent information about the five areas to be discussed here. Some general estimates are presented below. You may use them if you are unable to find the specific facts you need in the catalogs. If you have received any financial aid bulletins from the schools, read them carefully. Record any pertinent information. Since the figures in our estimates are based on data up to three years old, you will need to add another 8 to 10 percent per year since then to account for inflation. You will avoid disappointments by making your estimates a little on the high side.

Tuition and Special Fees

Tuition information can be found in the schools' catalogs under a section on enrollment, or tuition and fees. Special fees for services such as laboratories, health services, and student activities may be explained where these subjects are usually discussed in the catalog.

As a general rule, tuition and fees are lower at public institutions, particularly if you are a legal resident of the state or district in which the institution is located.

Books and Supplies

These costs vary only slightly with the type of institution. The amount relates to the type of course you select. Naturally, there will be more cost for art supplies for a student in an art institute. Courses in some academic areas require more books and more expensive books. Many professors now try to specify paperback versions of texts and required supplementary reading. Books at this writing may well cost a minimum of $30 a class unless you can buy them secondhand.

Room and Board

Institutions having on-campus housing usually report rates charged for room and board on a per-semester, per-quarter, or per-school-year basis. A small amount can sometimes be saved by finding off-campus housing and sharing it with several others. In general, off-campus housing costs about the same as living in a college dormitory.

Commuting students who live with their parents can save on room and board, but their expenses for daily transportation and for lunches and dinners at the school will somewhat offset the savings. In 1980 the College Entrance Examination Board estimated that the cost of room and board in a state university was $1,650 and suggested that money could be saved by commuters.

Personal Expenses

In the same College Board survey the expense of miscellaneous items such as wardrobe, soap, and toothpaste was estimated at $600.

Transportation

In planning your realistic college budget, be sure you include an estimate of transportation costs. If you plan to commute, consider the cost of a daily trip to the school and back. Multiply it by the number of school days.

If you plan to be a residential student, find out the cost of air or train fare, including transportation to and from the airport or train station. Most students make a total of three round trips per school year. This includes a trip home for the Christmas holidays and for spring vacation.

If you are a handicapped teenager with a mobility problem, you may need to figure an additional amount for on-campus transportation. This may be true for both commuting and residential students.

Once you have recorded all the information on the tally sheets, you can easily compare costs for attending the various schools. If you were unable to find all the information in the catalogs, you may need to write to the schools. Before you do, be sure you have jotted down any questions you may have about financial aid. You can include them in the same letter.

FOUR MAJOR SOURCES OF FUNDING

The four major sources of funding that should be checked out first are (1) the school itself; (2) the state vocational rehabilitation agency; (3) your own family; and (4) private sources, various clubs, industry, unions, etc. With luck, you may not have to go any further.

Funding Sources Administered by the School

The primary source for student assistance is the college, university, or business or technical school itself. Many institutions issue free publications about their student aid programs. If you have not received this literature from the schools you are seriously considering, send for it at once.

Many schools have considerable funds for scholarships. Many have been left to the school by alumni. Sometimes they are for special scholarships for special kinds of people, but often they are undesignated. The colleges usually have administrative control over this source of funding.

As a general rule, colleges also have loan funds. They also administer certain other federal grant and loan funds available to students.

The State-Federal Rehabilitation Agencies

Many handicapped persons are entitled to assistance from their state vocational rehabilitation agencies. These offices have been established to educate and train handicapped persons to achieve their potential in employment. The services that are provided include counseling and guidance, special education and training, and financial and other assistance while a person is receiving education and training. A list of state rehabilitation agencies appears in the Appendix.

Don't hesitate to ask your rehabilitation counselor for very specific services or programs. For example, if you want to pursue a particular career goal, you must ask for a specific type of assistance aimed at obtaining that objective (e.g., tuition assistance). Handicapped persons must not automatically assume that if the vocational rehabilitation agency (or counselor) does not mention a particular type of service, it is not available. Handicapped people should also question whether they are receiving the maximum amount of services and optimum benefit from programs offered by state vocational rehabilitation agencies.

During the last few years, programs have been established in every state to provide assistance to persons afflicted with developmental disabilities (e.g., mental retardation, cerebral palsy, epilepsy, and other similar conditions). Handicapped persons should contact their local vocational rehabilitation office, their state Developmental Disabilities Counsel, or both. Blind and visually handicapped persons should contact their state vocational agency for the blind.

Your rehabilitation counselor will know, or be willing to help you find, funding programs for which you qualify.

Your Family and Your Personal Resources

Most students attending a four-year institution make use of all four of the major sources. As you begin to get a clearer idea of just how much money you will need to attend the colleges on your preferred list, be sure you talk it over with your family. How much are they willing to contribute? How much do you think you will be able to earn? How much remains to be raised through other means? You and your family will be intimately involved with financing your education, no matter what combination of financial sources are put together. It is therefore important that you understand, at least in general, some of the many options for scholarships, fellowships, awards, grants, and loans and how one qualifies for them. The following is a brief summary of the many options.

SCHOLARSHIPS, FELLOWSHIPS, LOANS, AND GRANTS

About Scholarships

Many students start in their junior year in high school or even earlier to line up sources of scholarship money to finance their post-high school education. There are three types of scholarship awards—general, regional, and special.

General scholarships are available to qualified candidates regardless of residence, religion, sex, race, or field of study. The primary consideration is ability as measured by grades, rank in class, and various tests, plus financial need. There are also scholarships and contests that do not specify need as a prerequisite. Because of this absence of restriction, the competition for these funds is intense.

The National Merit Scholarships are well known and highly competitive. Need is not a basis for selection for the National Merit $1,000 and National Achievement $1,000 Scholarships. However, corporate-sponsored and college-sponsored National Merit and National Achievement Scholarships consider need in determining the amount of the scholarship awarded to each recipient. Academic competition determines the recipients of the scholarships.

Regional scholarships require recipients to be residents of certain localities. An example is the Hattie M. Strong Foundation, which awards loans to attend vocational schools only to residents of metropolitan Washington, D.C.

Special scholarships are offered by wide varieties of private organizations and individuals. They usually are limited to the interest areas that concern the organization or individual. Some are for persons of a certain ancestry or religion, place of employment, or vocational goal. Some are limited to the members of certain organizations, or to the children of members. Many financial aid officers or rehabilitation counselors are aware of only a small fraction of those that exist. So if you have need, it is worthwhile to check for scholarship funds with every organization to which you or your family belong. If you have a particular career goal, the trade association or professional association in that area may possibly help you locate scholarships.

If you apply for a scholarship, your family will have to reveal its financial circumstances. Your parents will be required to complete a detailed financial aid form. Based on this information, an estimate of the amount that your family could contribute yearly for your college education is calculated.

If you apply for financial aid in any form (scholarship, loan, or grant) from an institution or federal or state government, you will have to file a financial aid form. To be considered for the Pell Grant (previously known as the BEOG or Basic Educational Opportunity Grant) you must file a form. Addresses of some key places to obtain the forms are listed in the resources section. The Pell Grant program is a federal one. It is now tied in with other federal, state, and private programs. Be sure that you check with the school to which you are applying for aid, to learn which particular form or forms they require. Some state higher education agencies and private financial aid programs require that candidates apply for the Pell Grant. Thus it's a good idea to make application for Pell Grants early.

Current federal regulations require that handicapped students apply for Office of Education grant funds such as the Pell Grant before they apply to state vocational rehabilitation agencies for financial aid for college. Receipt of state vocational rehabilitation money is not dependent upon receipt of a Pell Grant.

About Loans

Loans are available from many sources—private foundations, organizations, businesses, clubs, service groups, state agencies, and the federal government.

Many communities now publish a *Directory of Student Aid,* which contains information about scholarships, loans, awards, and work-study opportunities. Your guidance counselor, the public library, the board of education, or the state department of education may be able to help you locate one for your area if it exists.

When you obtain loans, be certain that you know the terms of repayment, the interest rates, and what payments have to be made and when, while you are a student and after you leave or graduate.

The recent record of repayment of student loans has been not as high as expected. Some students receiving Guaranteed Student Loans have defaulted on their payments. By law, the schools and banks granting these loans are required to exert "due diligence" to obtain repayment. If the borrower is still in default after these efforts, the federal government will take steps to collect the debt. In most states a student aged eighteen or over has to sign a promissory note when obtaining the loan. This note makes the student legally obliged to repay the loan. He or she also will have to sign a repayment schedule. Whether educational loans are offered by private funds, colleges, or commercial organizations, you need to read the fine print and to understand the repayment conditions. Be sure you know exactly what you are letting yourself in for.

One lending group that has had a better than average repayment record on student educational loans is *United Student Aid Funds, Inc.,* which is a national, nonprofit corporation that endorses bank loans to college and graduate students. Usually the borrower deals with his home-town bank after receiving approval from his college or university. In New York, Manufacturers Hanover for over 40 years has helped finance students seeking higher education. For their student loan plan handbook, write NYSHESC, Student Information, Albany, NY 12255, or call, with questions, (800) 642-6234/6238.

FEDERAL FINANCIAL AID PROGRAMS

National Direct Student Loans (NDSL)

Most colleges and universities take part in the NDSL program. Loans are administered by various schools, colleges, and universities out of funds provided by the federal government and the institutions themselves.

Needy high school students who have been accepted for enrollment or post-secondary students enrolled at least half time as vocational, undergraduate, or graduate students are eligible to apply for NDSL loans.

If you are enrolled in a vocational program or if you have completed less than two years of a program leading to a bachelor's degree, you may borrow up to a total of $3,000. You may borrow up to $6,000 if you are an undergraduate student and have completed two years of study. This total includes the amount you borrowed under NDSL for your first two years of study. Graduate or professional students may borrow up to $12,000 under NDSL. This includes all NDSL amounts borrowed as an undergraduate.

Repayment begins six months after one graduates or leaves school for other reasons. The interest rate is 5 percent per year. Repayment may be extended over a ten-year period, with a minimum monthly payment of $30.

Guaranteed Student Loans (GSL)

Guaranteed loans are designed to make loan insurance available to any college student who wants to borrow money to help finance his or her education. These loans are primarily helpful to students from middle- and upper-income families who may not qualify for scholarships or NDSL loans. The student borrows directly from an approved bank or other financial institution. The loan is guaranteed by a state or a private nonprofit agency or by the federal government. The maximum amount that can be borrowed as an undergraduate is $2,500 a year. Total GSL debt for undergraduate and vocational students is $12,500; graduate and professional students, including loans made at undergraduate levels, $25,000. Repayment schedules are similar to those for NDSL, but the interest rate is 8 percent.

Pell Grants

This federally sponsored program provides grants to eligible full-time students and to high school graduates planning to attend college or other post-secondary institutions. Eligibility and amount of financial aid vary yearly. For the 1985–86 academic year, one can receive up to $2,000. This amount need not be paid back. You may obtain the necessary application forms from post-secondary educational institutions, high schools, state employment offices, or public libraries.

Supplemental Educational Opportunities Grants

This program provides for payment through post-secondary institutions to undergraduate or vocational students of exceptional financial need. High school students who have been accepted for at least half-time enrollment at an undergraduate or vocational school may also apply. Application forms and further information may be obtained from the director of financial aid at the institution in which you are or will be enrolled. The maximum amount of the grant is $2,000 per year. Again, because this is a grant, the money need not be paid back.

WORKING YOUR WAY THROUGH COLLEGE

Working your way through college is a well-honored American tradition. We have come a long way since the days when many college students sold magazine subscriptions or worked long hours in resort hotels in the summer. In winter they could usually be found working as waiters or waitresses or janitors in college dormitories, or at a variety of part-time jobs in stores and businesses in the college town. Since then the student's opportunities to earn money have been much expanded. If you plan to contribute some part toward the costs of your education, here in general are the options concerning summer jobs, part-time jobs, and work-study programs.

Part-time and Summer Jobs

Today in many schools, the majority of students are engaged in some sort of part-time work. Many colleges permit students to drop out to work full time for a year while they earn money to complete their education. The school's placement officers may help such students find jobs during their "earning leave" periods. They also help in finding part-time and summer work.

Most colleges place a limit on the number of hours a full-time student may work. This is usually from 10 to 20 hours a week. They usually suggest that you do not work during your freshman year while you adjust to college-level work and become accustomed to living away from home.

Income from your part-time job can be a part of the financial package that you and your family work out with the college financial aid officer, so talk to him or her about it.

College Work-Study Program

In an effort to provide students, especially those in the technical and professional fields, with experience in actual work situations, many colleges and universities have set up programs with business and industry in their vicinity. These cooperative work-study programs allow students to put into practice what they are studying in the classroom.

The College Work-Study Program of the Office of Education provides jobs for students who need financial aid and must earn a part of their educational expenses. The student must be enrolled at least half time as a vocational, undergraduate, or graduate student in an approved post-secondary institution. A participating institution arranges jobs on- or off-campus with a public or private nonprofit agency. As with other campus-based aid, the work-study award is set by the aid office at a limit that may not be exceeded. Thus, once you have received aid to the program's limit, you cannot continue to be employed under this program for the academic year.

The "co-op plan" may take different forms depending on the colleges and employees involved. In some, a full-time job is held by two students who alternate in work and study for specific periods of time throughout the school year. The more usual arrangement is that a student attends college full time for a quarter or a semester, then works full time for a quarter or a semester. This rotating pattern continues until graduation. The usual co-op work-study program leading to a bachelor's degree takes five years. For the student it has the inestimable value, as one educator phrased it, "of dipping him, at periodic intervals, into the reality of the world beyond the campus."

For the student who does not have a clear objective and who is seeking to orient himself or herself to the world of work, a series of assignments can be arranged to provide a breadth of experience.

For the student who has a clear career objective, the off-campus assignments provide sequences of work with increasing responsibility in his or her chosen field.

For the student with limited finances, earnings from cooperative assignments are a means of obtaining a college education that otherwise might be beyond his or her financial reach.

More than 900 colleges and universities in the U.S. and Canada have co-op education plans in operation. More colleges are planning to add them. A directory of two- and four-year institutions offering cooperative education plans is in the resources section.

CONCLUSION

Birdie Minor, the speech pathologist, got help through undergraduate school from the Department of Vocational Rehabilitation. She used some of her own savings and worked part time in summers. She also worked during one semester. She got a Rehabilitation Services Administration grant to go to graduate school.

June Stark is currently majoring in Italian at Georgetown University with the hope of going into foreign radio broadcasting. Most of her problems in financing her education were solved through the State Commission for the Blind, which allots funds for students in college. They even included extra money to cover fees for the necessary reading service.

Funds for his tuition to Temple University Medical School and a stipend for living costs came to *David Hartman* from the Bureau for the Visually Handicapped of Pennsylvania. Dr. Hartman became the first blind person ever to graduate from medical school. He is now serving his residency in psychiatry at a Philadelphia hospital.

From time to time we all read of special funds set up by a newspaper or radio station, usually for an accident victim. It is heartwarming to realize that, in these days of increasing lack of concern for our fellow

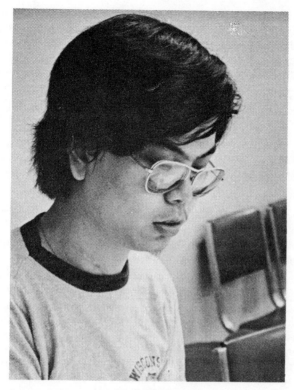

Paul Yeung

human beings, these fortunate people are the recipients of an outpouring of real concern shown by the generosity of the donors.

A Washington (D.C.) newspaper told the story of *Aron Had,* an artistically gifted Israeli who lost both hands in a war-related accident. The funds raised by the paper financed training in art at a local art institute.

Paul Yeung, paralyzed in an automobile accident while a student at the University of Wisconsin, has received fabulous amounts of help with his medical bills as well as his educational expenses. Many interested persons and organizations helped. These included a couple of appeals in the *Wisconsin Alumnus,* which goes to the university's thousands of graduates.

Doug Boyce was paralyzed after a wrestling accident while in high school. His friends pitched in not only to raise money but to raise his spirits and determination to go on living. They set up the Doug

Boyce Fund to help him pay his medical bills and get him started on his education. The fund pays the extras such as clothing and pocket money that are not covered by the State Rehabilitation Program, which pays his tuition.

It is true that only a very few will ever have a special fund set up for their education. However, you actually have many options.

As a handicapped person seeking to get a post-secondary education, you will face the same kind of financial hassle faced by everyone except the very rich. You have one additional source of funds that the nonhandicapped cannot use: the rehabilitation agencies. One thing is certainly clear. If you really want a post-high school education, there are many ways and means to finance it.

FINANCING-YOUR-EDUCATION CHECKLIST

For each of the schools to which you are applying for admission you should have:

1. Estimated the cost of attending per year.
2. Discussed your needs with your rehabilitation counselor to establish how much you may obtain from the Rehabilitation Agency.
3. Discussed your needs with your family and found out how much they may contribute.
4. Estimated whether you will be able to work for part of the needed expenses.
5. Discussed your needs with the financial aid officers of the schools.
6. If necessary, applied for scholarships, fellowships, or loans:

   as recommended by financial aid officers;
   as located through membership organizations to which your family belongs.

7. Checked through the resources section to see if you have forgotten to take any necessary steps.
8. Sent in your applications for admission and for other financial aids as needed.

When all the replies are in, make your choice and follow up with the needed steps to prepare yourself for entry. It is courteous, after you are all set to attend one specific school, to advise the other schools that you will not be attending.

SELECTED RESOURCES CHAPTER IV— FINANCING YOUR EDUCATION

Notes: Information has been listed as much as possible in the order in which the subjects were discussed in the preceding chapter.

Some listed publications are free, some cost a little, and some are expensive. Ask the price, or include a line saying "Send only if it costs less than $1.00 or $5.00" or whatever.

* indicates books that can usually be found in public libraries or in your guidance or rehabilitation counselor's office.

COLLEGE COSTS

The College Cost Book, College Entrance Examination Board, College Board Publications Orders, Box 2815, Princeton, NJ 08504.

Meeting College Costs. College Scholarship Service, 888 7th Avenue, New York, NY 10019. Copies should be available in high school guidance offices.

SOME MAJOR RESOURCES FOR SEEKING STUDENT FINANCIAL AID

* *Scholarships, Fellowships and Loans, Vol. VI,* 1977. Bellman Publishing Company, P.O. Box 164, Arlington, MA 02174. This book is considered the standard reference guide in the field.

Scholarships, Fellowships and Loans News Service, published quarterly. Bellman Publishing Company. Address above.

Don't Miss Out. The Ambitious Student's Guide to Scholarships and Loans, 1985–86, 9th ed. Octameron Associates, P.O. Box 3437, Alexandria, VA 22302.

Handicapped Funding Directory, A Guide to Sources of Funding in the U.S. for Handicapped Programs and Services, 1982–83, 3d ed. Research Grant Guides, P.O. Box 357, Oceanside, NY 11572.

The As and Bs of Academic Scholarships, A Guide to Current Programs, 1985–86, 7th ed. Octameron Associates, address above.

Student Aid Bulletin. Chronicle Guidance Publications, Inc. Morovia, NY 13118. Lists scholarships available in each state.

AID FROM PRIVATE ORGANIZATIONS

Businesses

Thousands of programs are available from concerns for which the parents or the students themselves work. Many also make funds available on a competitive basis to students preparing for certain careers for which the industry has a need. The trade or professional association for a given industry can usually tell you if anything is available.

Many businesses also grant tuition refunds through a special educational plan. A company may pay full tuition or pay only for part of a single course.

Labor Unions

Many labor unions now have scholarships, fellowships, or loans available primarily to members or children of members. Some of this aid is given as prizes for winning contests. Students should inquire of their parents' unions.

Scholarships. AFL-CIO, 815 16th Street, NW, Room 47, Washington, DC 20006. A useful guide for meeting college expenses.

Religious Groups

National agencies sponsored by various faiths have local and national information on student assistance, as do many clergymen. There are a number of funds that provide student assistance to people of various faiths. Your temple, church, or synagogue may be able to help you find financial aid.

Other Membership Organizations

Need a Lift?. American Legion Education and Scholarship Program, Box 1055, Indianapolis, IN 46206. A gold mine of information on student aid from all sources for veterans, their dependents, and nonveterans. It contains a summary of scholarships and loans sponsored by individual states.

Students in need should check out all the organizations to which anyone in the family belongs including trade and professional, religious, and fraternal organizations.

Winning Contests

Gadney's Guide to 1800 International Contests, Festivals and Grants in Film and Video, Photography, TV-Radio Broadcasting, Writing, Poetry and Playwriting, Journalism; rev. ed. 1980. Festival Publications, P.O. Box 10180, Glendale, CA 19209.

The National Association of Secondary School Principals puts out a yearly list of educational contests. Not all of these offer scholarships as prizes. To obtain a copy, write to the National Association of Secondary School Principals, 1904 Associations Drive, Reston, VA 22091.

Contests provide an opportunity for you to test your talents and abilities in competitive situations. Local newspapers often list names of winners. By following the papers early in high school you can accumulate a list of local contests.

Many administrators of private scholarship funds require you to write an essay on your educational and vocational plans. They give preference to able writers who show a breadth of interests.

AID FROM STATE AND LOCAL GOVERNMENTS

Departments of Education

State departments of education usually supply information on student aid available in their own state. Many states have higher education assistance corporations that aid many thousands of students.

Write to the state department of education to locate a state scholarship directory. When available, these often list scholarships, fellowships, and work-study programs available in your state.

Local Governments and Newspapers

Local financial aid directories are occasionally compiled. Check with your guidance counselor or call the mayor's office to see what you can find out.

Local scholarships are often announced in local papers or magazines. Trade and professional publications also often note the existence of scholarships.

AID FROM THE FEDERAL GOVERNMENT

Members of Congress

Senators and Congressmen can be helpful to parents, counselors, and students. They will furnish copies of the latest student aid materials available through the U.S. government.

U.S. Department of Education

One way to find out about the programs administered by the Department of Education is through your state and local rehabilitation centers; see the Appendix.

For the U.S. Department of Education's "Student Guide" write to the Federal Student Aid Program, P.O. Box 84, Washington, DC 20044. This pamphlet lists the state agencies for the Guaranteed Student Loan program and describes other available loan and aid programs.

Federal Student Aid Information Center, P.O. Box 4150, Iowa City, Iowa 52244, or call (301) 984-4070 with specific questions.

Veterans Administration

The best-known program is the GI Bill, under which funds are paid directly to eligible students to finance college, graduate, or vocational study. You must have served more than 180 days on active duty, part of which occurred after January 31, 1955, and before January 1, 1977, or have been released after January 31, 1955, for a service-connected disability. For information, send for the booklet *Federal Benefits for Veterans and Dependents* (VA IS-1 Fact Sheet). Superintendent of Documents, U.S. Government Printing Office, Washington, DC 20402. This is updated from time to time.

Children and spouses of veterans whose death or total, permanent disability were service-connected, and of service persons missing in action or prisoners of war are eligible for training and educational benefits.

Some states have benefits for children and spouses of deceased or disabled veterans. Check the veterans department of the state in which you are currently living and the state in which your parents lived at the time the veteran parent entered service or became disabled or died.

PART-TIME JOBS AND CO-OP WORK PLANS

1985 Summer Employment Directory: Where the Jobs Are and How to Get Them, 34th ed. Writer's Digest Books, 9933 Alliance Rd., Cincinnati, Ohio 45242. Lists summer jobs state by state.

The Job Sharing Handbook, by Barney Olmsted & Suzanne Smith, 1983. Penguin Books, 625 Madison Avenue, New York, NY.

Moonlighting: A Complete Guide to Over 200 Exciting Part-time Jobs, by Peter Davidson. McGraw Hill Book Co. 1983.

For a complete list of two- and four-year institutions offering cooperative education programs, write to the National Commission for Cooperative Education, 360 Huntington Avenue, Boston, MA 02115.

TO OBTAIN FORMS TO FILE FOR FINANCIAL, EDUCATIONAL AID

Family Financial Statement (FFS) distributed by the American College Testing Program (ACT). P.O. Box 1000, Iowa City, IA 52240.

Financial Aid Form (FAF) distributed by the College Scholarship Service (CSS), Princeton, NJ 08540.

Pennsylvania Higher Assistance Agency Form (PHEAA), Towne House, Harrisburg, PA 17102.

For application determination of the Federal Pell Grant both the FFS and the FAF are applicable.

CHAPTER V

Finding the Right Job and Career

If you are presently grappling with the problem of deciding upon a career area, selecting a school, or financing your education, you are probably several months or years away from seeking your first job in your chosen field. Nevertheless, since your career choice is so closely related to this, we would like to present a brief survey of what may be involved. In addition to applying for and obtaining your first job after you finish your training, it should help you obtain any part-time or summer work you need in the more immediate future.

Finding your first full-time job is not easy for any young person whether he or she is handicapped or not. Everyone has to deal with that bugaboo of not being accepted for employment because he or she has no previous experience, but not being able to get a job prevents you from gaining the experience. Certain additional problems are faced by nearly every handicapped person. Here are some examples:

Some years ago when *Dr. Robert Menchel,* senior physicist with the Xerox Corporation, launched his search for a job, sixty-two employers rejected his application. This was during a period when the technical job market was booming. One application even came back to him with a notation that the company did not hire deaf people. Legislation passed in 1973 prevents discrimination against handicapped people; yet much of the old attitude remains. Dr. Menchel said that potential employers focused mainly on his handicap and did not give his qualifications first priority.

Dr. David Hartman, who dislikes being referred to as a blind physician, got his first job when he was in high school. He and a buddy attended a camp. In the second year his buddy was put on the paid staff while he was asked to do the same work as a volunteer. "What

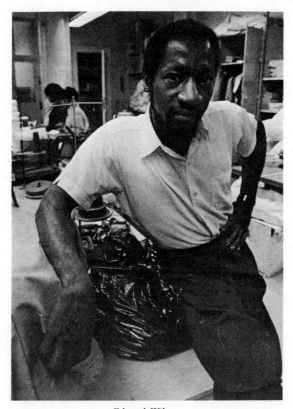

Edward Wilson

bothers me," says Dr. Hartman in his recent book *White Coat, White Cane,* "was that a sighted person would get the job first, then go on to prove his or her competence or the lack of it—the risk was the employer's. The blind person, on the other hand, always has to prove himself first."

Jo Ann Haseltine, federal office worker, says, "Although the rules and regulations say it is against the law to discriminate against handicapped people when applying for jobs, I know that law is not very well enforced. When I first started federal service, I had to change jobs from time to time, usually because of reduction in force situations. I would never tell the new employer about my disabilities (she is learning-disabled) until after they had hired me. I tried telling and laying my cards on the table but soon found out that I didn't get the job."

Edward Wilson, an employee of Mt. Sinai Hospital who has epilepsy, agrees with Jo Ann. "Employers didn't inquire into my medical history, and I didn't tell them about my attacks." Wilson considers himself lucky because he has never lost a job because of epilepsy. Many employers fire people with this disease after an on-the-job attack.

Dennis Smith, who received a medical discharge from the Navy because of epilepsy, speaks of the problems he faced in finding a job. "After being unemployed for a while, and being rejected from jobs you're qualified for, you begin to feel negative about yourself. You get vibes from employers and start thinking maybe they're right."

Lina Padilla, a native of the Philippines who lives in the United States, was stricken with polio when she was four. She began her job search when she burst out of a highly protected home environment. With the help of two Peace Corps friends, she went around the world, wheelchair and all. "You soon learn that you're at the bottom of the employment list," says Lina. "I remember when I was in business school, I was often last to be hired for temporary jobs." Lina now works for the National Education Association in Washington, D.C. She has held several other jobs and interviewed for countless others. She believes she got her first full-time job as a secretary with an insurance company in part because the man she worked for was also in a wheelchair. When her applications were not accepted, it has often been because the employer made his own judgment of whether she would or could get to work and whether she would be dependable. As Dr. Hartman has also discovered, the handicapped person has to prove that he or she can do the job, and often doesn't get the chance to do that.

The important thing to remember about these people, as well as all the others mentioned in previous chapters, is not that they had problems. It is that they solved the problems. The truth is that most young people who want to work will somehow manage to overcome the obstacles and go on to rewarding careers.

SOME BARRIERS YOU MAY ENCOUNTER

Much progress has been made in recent years toward integrating handicapped people fully into the mainstream of society. As a handicapped person about to move into the world of work, you need to understand the barriers that remain so that you can cope with them. Barriers not only pose problems for getting a job, but they exist in every aspect of your work life and your life-style. Your specific legal rights as they relate to barriers will be discussed in the next chapter.

There are four main types of barriers: architectural, transportation, attitudinal, and bureaucratic.

Architectural Barriers

Much progress has been made in overcoming architectural barriers since the Easter Seal Society started the Architectural Barriers Program in 1945. Publicity picturing a person in a wheelchair at the foot of a hopelessly long flight of stairs has begun to make inroads on the ignorance and indifference of the public. Yet today some buildings are still being built that are inaccessible. Federal legislation can control only building projects that receive federal funding.

A common architectural barrier for a handicapped applicant is to find that the particular building or office is inaccessible. It may have an accessible entrance but inaccessible storage areas or washrooms. Under the new laws an employer cannot discriminate against you because you are handicapped. He or she is required to make such architectural modifications as are necessary for you to work. Yet it is not always possible for suitable arrangements to be made at the time the need presents itself.

Transportation Barriers

The plight of blind people who are routinely deprived of their canes while in airplanes is certainly an example of a transportation barrier to the blind. Airlines still make some seemingly unreasonable regulations about the number and kinds of handicapped persons who may obtain passage on any given flight. They sometimes require an attendant or companion to travel with the handicapped person. Subway systems are being built with escalators and only a single, often hidden elevator to serve persons in wheelchairs. These are just a few of the transportation barriers that remain. This is in spite of the fact that you may have solved any individual problems you have relating to getting around.

Rehabilitation legislation was passed in the 1970s for a new, fully accessible transbus system. The idea was that as cities needed to replace old buses in their systems, they would be required to replace them with transbuses (buses with a floor height of 22 inches instead of 36 inches). However, this project was abandoned in 1979.

Since 1979, federal regulations require that each transit authority in the country use its federal funds in one of three ways to provide accessibility for the handicapped. Transit authorities may purchase lifts to make the existing system accessible; they may purchase new Power Transit Vans, which are specialized vans with lifts; or they may choose to implement a combination of the two.

This use of federal funds works well or does not, depending on where you live. For instance, New York City in 1985 had 1,887 buses with lifts, or 48 percent of the buses, making buses relatively accessible to the handicapped in the city. If you know the schedules, you can get a bus. On the other hand, in Philadelphia, where Power Transit Vans are used, it is estimated that the vans make only 600 trips a day, denying service to a large percentage of the handicapped population.

The Power Transit Vans are operating cost-intensive because of the fees paid to drivers, gas expenses, and so on. The buses with lifts may have a high initial capital cost, but the money is earned back from bus fares and usage.

Check with your transit authority to find out what kind of program it has implemented, and then apply for the half-fare cards that are offered by most transit authorities in the country.

Communications Barriers

Many deaf, blind, and learning-disabled persons suffer from communications barriers. For information on what is being done, write to National Center for a Barrier Free Environment (see resources section).

Attitudinal Barriers

One of the authors, who was a weak and undersized child because of a heart defect, still cringes when she remembers how her best friend's mother used to refer to her as "poor little Norma!" It stiffened her determination to prove just the opposite. Handicapped people hate to be labeled by their handicap or classified in any way they regard as belittling. They feel that the label never exactly fits, and usually it does not.

As *Virginia Meyers* explains, "Being retarded means it's twice as hard showing people how we are, that we can live like normal people. We're not that dumb; we're slow-minded is all." Virginia is the wife of *Roger Meyers* and one of the two principal characters in Robert Meyers' book *Like Normal People* (McGraw Hill, 1978). The book is the true story of his family's struggle for a normal life for his retarded brother Roger. A newer term being used these days is "the intellectually impaired," but that is just a different label.

Labeling people presents a paradox. How can we pass laws and provide special benefits for certain kinds of people without labeling and classifying them? Yet placing a label on someone, no matter how honestly or how conscientiously it is done, is often the first step toward forming a stereotype.

A dictionary definition of "stereotype" is "a conventional, formulaic, and usually oversimplified conception, opinion, or belief." Stereotyping is one of fourteen attitudinal barriers being studied by the *Regional Rehabilitation Research Institute on Attitudinal, Legal and Leisure Barriers.* The institute is affiliated with George Washington University in Washington, D.C. The other barriers are prejudice, ignorance, fear, insensitivity, bigotry, misconception, discrimination, dislike, invisibility, discomfort, condescension, and intolerance. The institute defines attitudinal barriers as "a way of thinking or feeling resulting in behavior that limits the potential of disabled people to be independent individuals." The following story illustrates a barrier due to a misconception. It is taken from one of the institute's publications.

"Mark, a paraplegic in a wheelchair, is seated in a restaurant with his wife, Ann. The waitress comes to take their order and asks Ann, 'What would he like to order?' " The waitress' attitude reflects her belief that since Mark is in a wheelchair he is helpless and unable to order his own dinner. Such situations may be complicated by the fact that the waitress feels uncomfortable with Mark and his chair.

Misconceptions or the lack of knowledge lead some employers to make wrong assumptions about the capabilities of handicapped people. It is the most common barrier faced by a disabled job seeker. Because the employer cannot imagine how he himself could do the job from a wheel chair, wearing braces, not being able to see, or whatever, he assumes that a handicapped applicant (you) cannot do it. These problems are compounded by the fact that many nonhandicapped people are half afraid of handicapped people. They are distinctly uncomfortable with them and do not know how to treat them.

Bureaucratic Barriers

If you or your family have had to deal with a state rehabilitation agency to obtain services to which you are entitled, you may already know about red tape. One must be prepared for a lot of waiting, a lot of filling out of forms, and a lot of just plain frustration. It seems to be the price one pays for receiving what is due from any government agency. Many examples of bureaucratic problems and delays were described in the discussion of the fate of the transbus.

Dr. David Hartman, and Temple University School of Medicine where he trained, both experienced frustrations over the erratic and belated way that the agency sent his tuition and living stipend payments. Before that, Hartman had to deal with the innumerable bureaucracies in medical schools that couldn't imagine how a blind person might become a physician. They rejected his application in spite of his superior qualifications.

Robert Meyers in his book *Like Normal People* summed up the problem and the disappointments. "The existence of laws, legislative programs, Presidential decrees, and funding that made Roger's residence at the facility possible does not mean the end of his problem. . . . A bureaucratic morass has been created among federal, state and local authorities, and competing agencies within each of those jurisdictions, which does not always work to the advantage of retarded people."

Coping with the bureaucracy has become a way of life for most Americans. Even the smallest wage earner who files his short-form income tax return is not immune from possible problems with the Internal Revenue Service. Says Robert Meyers in an earlier part of his book, "State funds for such fees [to pay for a residential facility for Roger] were available for the first time under legislation signed by President Kennedy—a sign of the changing times. But it is an imperfect world, and red tape prevented my parents from gaining access to them."

To cope successfully with the bureaucracy you need to be persistent and never, never give up. *Keith Heuer,* a double amputee, has been fighting the bureaucracy for a long time and has recently won his latest battle. This is his story.

Keith was well under way with a successful career in the Navy when he lost his legs in an automobile accident in 1967. The Navy was a particularly good career choice—since childhood he had spent much of his time working around or aboard boats—but the accident put an end to Keith's Navy career. He realized, however, that whatever he did with the rest of his life would have to involve boats.

Keith followed the usual recovery and rehabilitation routine. The Navy fitted him with artificial legs that brought him up to his usual height of over six feet. But he discovered that he couldn't maneuver around a ship on the rolling sea as well as he had before. So he devised what he calls "stubbies," prostheses fitted directly over the stumps of his legs. Wearing "stubbies" he is 4'6" tall. Once more he was able to walk the decks even when the sea was rough, climb ladders, and hoist himself to the helmsman's seat. In fact, his new shorter body structure is more stable in some ways.

For eight years after the accident, Keith handled a number of jobs. He piloted boats for other owners. He served as mate aboard a succession of oceangoing motor vessels. Gradually he defined his new career goal— to own and operate his own boating business. To do this he needed to become a licensed passenger ship captain. He operated his own boat for a while after obtaining a Panamanian license. The Coast Guard didn't recognize this license, so in 1975 Keith began his struggle to obtain a U.S. captain's license. He sent in his application to the Coast Guard, along with required documents to certify his competence and experience. He was told he was "disabled," "not mobile," and "too short to see over the helm." Most of his qualifications were rejected, including the needed years of experience at sea.

Coast Guard bureaucrats seemed to operate on a very simple logic:

Only ablebodied persons can be licensed ship captains.
Keith Heuer is disabled by reason of having lost part of each leg.
Therefore, Keith Heuer should be denied a captain's license.

All judgments were made from the application form and supporting documents supplied by the applicant. On paper, Keith was "disabled." The question of whether he could do the job in spite of this never seems to have come up. They were most reluctant to allow him a chance to prove whether he could do the job or not.

He volunteered to take a physical examination. The doctors found him "competent." Finally, after more time and more pressure, officials agreed to test his abilities. Coast Guard officials watched as Keith operated the boat. He passed the test. This bureaucratic change of heart was probably due in part to the fact that ABC Television gave a lot of publicity to Keith's story. They showed him scampering up and down ladders, operating a helmsman's console, and literally swarming all over the boat.

But the battle was not over. The bureaucracy lost some important papers accompanying Steve's application. They asked for additional documentation, some of it impossible to obtain, and verifications from men now deceased. When the license finally came it contained unworkable restrictions. Keith would be permitted to operate the boat only in daylight hours, and then only with another licensed operator aboard.

Keith has spent more than $4,000 on his battle for a license. This was not his first encounter with bureaucracy. He first met resistance of the medical bureaucracy when he decided that the best course for him would be to dispense with his artificial legs. The medical and rehabilitation people tried to talk him out of it. Later when he and his business partner tried to get a loan from the Small Business Administration, they had to try no less than five times.

The battle for a license has been won, however. A follow-up television program reported that the Coast Guard had reevaluated Keith's sea-duty time and given him credit for almost all the days required. He took the written examination for his captain's license, passed it, and received his license in July, 1979.

LETTERS AND RÉSUMÉS

Before you go out to acquire your first professional job you will need to acquire some know-how for writing application letters, drawing up résumés, and conducting yourself at interviews. Just as you began to plan your higher education while you were still in high school, you should begin to plan your campaign for your first job during your college years.

Many schools and colleges hold career recruitment sessions. During these, representatives from business visit the campus to interview prospective employees. In most schools such sessions are scheduled by the placement or employment office. Schedule yourself for as many interviews as you can. Although such early interviews may not lead directly to employment, they can give you needed experience in handling yourself in the interview situation. Persons in the placement office or office for student personnel services are also often able to help you design effective résumés, write application letters, and find possible job openings.

In a book this size we cannot go very far into detail on how to find a job. Some suggestions for good books will be found in the resources section. Rather, we shall make a few suggestions on writing résumés and application letters, and on job interviews. We shall discuss some of the issues that may arise because of your disability.

Writing Your Résumé

Writing your résumé is an excellent exercise in organizing your thinking. It opens the door for many jobs. You can learn how to present your achievements in life in the most effective order. After all, that is what you have to sell an employer. Katherine Nash, successful career counselor, defines résumé in her book *Get the Best of Yourself:* "It is a concise account of your experiences and qualifications as an applicant for a position. It tells something of your experiences and qualifications and professional background, and since it is distributed among prospective employers, it presumably relates to a job." She says it should be "a record of your vocational successes." In the case of young people with little or no work experience, it can be a record of success in handling problems and situations similar to those that might be encountered in the sought-after job.

You will probably be ahead of the game if you begin early in your college years to think about what to put down on your own personal "record of success." Then when you need to write a résumé, you can select the best from among items you might otherwise have forgotten.

When you get to the point of actually needing a résumé, you will quickly discover that one basic résumé is rarely suitable for many different job situations. Once you have organized the basic material, you will find it easier to pull together what you need for a particular job interview.

One question may come to mind. "Do I have to include my failures as well as my successes?" Maybe you were fired last year from your job at the college bookstore. What about that?

Katherine Nash says you don't have to include failures because "You're not applying for a position you expect to fail at so why hobble your hopes with a recollection of past frustrations?" She doesn't think it's dishonest either. The employer will not be hiring you for the things you cannot do, but for what you can do. Of course, if this leaves a noticeable time gap in your résumé, and if the employer should ask you about it, the best policy is to tell the truth. That way you will have a chance to explain the circumstances. You would not have such an opportunity if you had entered it on your résumé. And of course, the subject may never come up.

We agree that the best policy is to tell the truth, but how much, if anything, should you say about your disability? Before you decide, there is one helpful question you can answer for yourself: "Does the prospective employer need to be alerted that I am handicapped so that it does not come as a shock when I go for an interview?"

Persons with invisible handicaps like epilepsy, retardation, or learning disabilities frequently choose not to say anything about it in their résumés, application letters, or interviews. They reason that by the time it becomes necessary for the boss to know about the disability, the employee will have had a chance to prove that he or she can do the job. Explanations can be made more satisfactorily at that time.

Persons with highly visible handicaps do not have this choice. They must prepare future employers. One place to put this in your résumé is in the section on personal information. Many people include such items as height, weight, age and marital status, and general health. Skip a space so that your disability will not be confused with your health. Enter the name of your disability. Follow this with a short statement of the ways in which you compensate.

For example, *Orlo Nichols* is a blind actuary who works for the Social Security Administration in Baltimore. He found that employers cannot imagine how a blind man could handle such work. Orlo was rejected by a number of employers in spite of his excellent qualifications. He might have allayed the worst worries of potential employers if his résumé had said something like this:

Personal

Age: 37
Marital status: Married, 2 children
Health: Excellent

Disability: Blind since birth; able to handle communications efficiently with aid of typewriter, dictating machine, telephone, braille calculator, keypunch machine, and opticon. Occasionally employ a reader.

Even if the potential employer doesn't know what some of the pieces of equipment are, it opens his mind to the fact that there are many ways in which a blind person compensates.

The National Paraplegia Foundation, in a booklet on "Preparing Yourself to Go to Work," recommends that a somewhat more detailed statement of "physical condition" be included in the résumé, and that the résumé be included in all letters to potential employers.

According to one employment counselor, an average employer will give a résumé a five- to ten-second scan. This is true whether it is included with your letter or presented at the time of the interview. Try to write something brief that emphasizes the points you want emphasized. Never send out a résumé unaccompanied by a letter.

Only you can decide what and how much you should say about your handicap in your résumé. Be sure to talk it over with your career counselor. Discuss it with your rehabilitation counselor. His or her special knowledge of the experiences of other handicapped people may be of value to you.

Writing Letters

The main purpose of writing to a potential employer is not to apply for a job. It is not even to ask for an application blank. It is, according to Katherine Nash and other career counselors, to motivate the employer to invite you to come in for an interview. To include a copy of your résumé with this first contact letter may weigh it down with too much information too soon. Usually it is better to drop a few hints as to how your abilities might fit his needs and to express a genuine interest in the company.

If you are not including a résumé with your letter but still feel a need to alert the potential employer to your disability, you need to work into the letter the information in the disability statement from your résumé. You must consider the fact that the reader may be distracted from your whole carefully constructed sequence of thought designed to motivate him or her to invite you in for an interview. If you handle the explanation subtly, however, it may increase the employer's interest in meeting you personally. The best of all situations is when you can say that So-and-So recommended that you write to the employer. It is A-OK when you can depend on So-and-So to have mentioned to the employer that you are handicapped. It can then be left out of the letter.

Here again, it is a good idea to discuss your letter with your placement counselor or your rehabilitation counselor.

JOB INTERVIEWS

The purpose of the job interview from an employer's point of view is to give him or her a chance to evaluate you as a potential member of his team of employees. The employer wants to find out if you would contribute to or improve the enterprise in which the company is engaged. From your own point of view, the purpose is usually to impress on the employer that you are willing and able to make such a contribution. This puts the employer and you in a somewhat adversarial relationship. The employer looks for reasons why you can do the job, but he is also evaluating reasons why you cannot. You, the applicant, are stuck with the dreary task of "proving" you can do a job that you know much less about than the employer does.

Your mental attitude to interviews will be greatly improved if you think of them as mutual evaluation sessions. You are just as interested in evaluating the employer and the company as he or she is in finding out if you can do the job. One young person we know comforts herself with the philosophy that there is only one *right* place for her to work at any given time in her life. During the interview, it usually becomes apparent to her whether that company is the right place or not.

Career counselors agree that there are several basic things that are important to consider in approaching a job interview. They are summed up in the popular maxims "Be prepared" and "Put your best foot forward."

Be Prepared

Once you have been invited to come in for an interview, there is still much you can do to prepare yourself. Here are a few suggestions.

1. Learn all you can about the company. Read carefully any literature that has been sent to you. Keep your eyes open for reports in newsmagazines and newspapers that relate to the company or the industry. Spend some time in the library periodical room to cover recent business publications you do not ordinarily see. Look up the company in some of the directories put out by leading business publications. You might find information on the officers of the company in *Who's Who in America*. You may or may not have an opportunity

to mention any of this, but it will give you a more confident basis for the interview.

2. Study your résumé with the employer's requirements for the job in mind. Be prepared to explain how one or several of your specific qualifications match specific needs of the job.

3. Prepare two question lists. The first consists of a few simple questions. Ask about what you need to know to decide whether this is the right place for you to work. Mentally outline your ideal working place. Design the questions to find out how many of these qualities the company has. Do not bring up the salary question at this point in the interview. Ask questions on the things that are important to you as a person.

The second question list is made up of intelligent questions that have come to mind as you did your research on the company. A question is an inoffensive way to take the initiative in an interview situation. A question on the subject under discussion can frequently be inserted. A question is often appreciated because it can reflect your knowledge of the company and your interest in the job. Of course, if you are being interviewed by the number one company in the industry and you ask, "Oh, by the way, is this a big company?" it will not help you much. Your questions must be intelligent ones.

A third kind of question, or at least topic for conversation, is about the profession. If you are talking about engineering, for example, what you say about engineering will reflect your education and background in the field.

4. The employer may introduce the salary question by asking what are your minimum salary requirements. This puts you on the spot. If you name too large a figure, you may be ruled out of the position altogether. If you name too small a figure, the employer may be glad to hire you at that figure. You will then be stuck with a smaller salary than you might otherwise have negotiated. How can one avoid falling into this trap? Most advertised positions, or ones listed with placement agencies, give a salary range. That is your starting point. It gives you an idea of what the job is worth to the company. The upper level usually represents what they would be willing to pay an exceptionally qualified and experienced applicant. The lower levels represent what they are willing to pay for an inexperienced but well trained and educated applicant. Don't start with the very bottom rate you are prepared to accept. Remember, it is always easier to move down to a smaller figure than to move up. It usually makes points also to say that you are willing to start at a lower figure for a trial period while you are learning the job and proving your value to the employer.

Putting Your Best Foot Forward

Your general appearance is important. What you wear to the interview communicates something to everyone who sees you. If you don't believe this, spend an afternoon in the park. Draw mental character sketches of every person you see. Perhaps you will see a girl in frayed jeans, a fellow in muddy boots and a hard hat, a woman in a business suit, a woman in a frilly dress wearing a pillbox hat, a man in a vested, navy blue suit. The mental images you form are drawn in part from the person's demeanor. More important, they are drawn from observing his or her clothing.

Be sure the clothes you wear to the interview give the message you want them to give—even if this means you have to borrow something. One good rule of thumb is to wear something similar to what is being worn by persons now working for the company on the grade level of the position you are seeking. It is important that you feel comfortable in the clothes you are wearing.

An employment counselor who appeared recently on TV gave these basic rules that may be applied if you are seeking employment in an office or a profession.

1. *Don't dress too casually.* For women this means a skirt and sweater and sandals are too casual. For men, a loud plaid sports jacket or leisure suit is too casual.

2. *Women should not wear mannish styles.* The vogue for pants suits in business seems to be declining. Skirts seem to command more respect.

3. *The ideal outfit for a job interview* should be well coordinated and "give the impression you are well pulled together." For women this means a skirt, jacket, and blouse not too extreme in design, pattern, or color. It means a minimum of tasteful jewelry—nothing that calls attention to itself like clanking bracelets. For men this means a business suit, a white or pastel shirt, and a tie that is not too flashy.

Be sure to discuss up-coming interviews, including what to wear, with your placement counselor or rehabilitation counselor.

CONCLUSION

More and more employers are coming to understand disabled people. They are beginning to recognize that disabled teenagers can make valuable contributions. Among them are E. I. du Pont de Nemours & Co., McDonnell Douglas Corporation, Sears, Roebuck and Company, National Restaurant Association/Food Services Industry, Tennessee Valley Authority, International Business Machines, and Consolidated Edison. Many of these companies not only promote the hiring of persons with handicaps but also provide in-house rehabilitation services and special placement programs.

Du Pont, for example, in the decade 1973–1982 increased its handicapped population by 89 percent, from 1,452 to 2,745 employees. During the same period the total number of Du Pont employees increased by only 13 percent. A survey of handicapped employees revealed them to be safe, productive, and dependable. Supervisors were asked to rate handicapped employees and to make a peer comparison using a sample of nonimpaired employees. In safety, 96 percent of the handicapped were rated average or above average, compared with 92 percent for nonimpaired employees. In performance of job duties, the handicapped improved their rating slightly from the survey of 1973, recording 92 percent average or above, compared with 91 percent for nonimpaired employees. A measurable improvement was noted in the area of attendance, with handicapped employees rated average or above rising from 79 percent in 1973 to 85 percent, compared with 91 percent for nonimpaired employees. Du Pont is also active in working with the community in such projects as sheltered workshops for severly handicapped persons who may never be able to work in industry, and vocational rehabilitation centers that train handicapped people to enter or reenter the work force.

An encouraging story appeared in *Boardroom Reports,* a monthly magazine for top management and board members. It showed that the courts are working well to aid in the implementation of the new legislation on behalf of the disabled. *Boardroom Reports* listed these recent court decisions:

- A school board was held to have violated the law by refusing to hire a blind teacher. Court's reasoning: classroom assignment could have been arranged to accommodate her needs.
- A diabetic could not be assumed to be incapable of controlling the condition and being a productive worker.
- A one-eyed employee was entitled to the job even though his disability prevented him from reading fine print.
- A taxi company violated the law by barring a one-armed applicant. Reason: a slight modification of the steering wheel made it easy for him to drive well, and his record was free of chargeable accidents.
- A company did not have the right to exclude an employee solely because of a degenerative disease that was likely to make him unemployable in a few years.

The world is never perfect. It may not be the best of all possible times to be a handicapped person, but it certainly is a lot better than it used to be.

SELECTED RESOURCES CHAPTER V—FINDING A JOB

Notes: Information has been listed in this section in the order the subjects were discussed earlier in the chapter.

Some listed publications are free, some cost a little, and some are expensive. Ask the price, or include a line saying "Send only if it costs less than $1.00, or $5.00" or whatever.

*indicates books that can usually be found in public libraries or in your guidance or rehabilitation counselor's office.

BARRIERS IN GENERAL

National Center for a Barrier Free Environment, Access Center, 1140 Connecticut Avenue, NW, Suite 1006, Washington, DC 20036. Directs programs and research on barriers and publishes a report. Distributes publications on barrier-free design.

National Easter Seal Society for Crippled Children and Adults, 2023 West Ogden Avenue, Chicago, IL 60612. This society also does much work on developing barrier-free design and has many publications directed toward architects and other professionals.

Attitudinal Barriers

The Regional Rehabilitation Research Institute on Attitudinal, Legal and Leisure Barriers, 1828 L St., NW, Suite 704, Washington, DC 20036. Has many publications. The following two are part of a series. Write for a publications list.

The Invisible Battle—Attitudes Toward Disability; 15 pages. (address above)
Counterpoint; 15 pages. (address above)

Architectural Barriers

Architectural and Transportation Barriers Compliance Board, Washington, DC 20201. This board is the authority on compliance with the law as it relates to architectural barriers relating to facilities used in programs that receive federal funding and on all federal buildings and programs. Write for specific information.

Communications Barriers

Societies serving the deaf, the blind, the learning-disabled, and others have studied the special problems of communications barriers in those areas. For a list of national agencies, see the Appendix.

Bureaucratic Barriers

Organizations set up to work for the civil and legal rights of handicapped people often can help you find ways to cope with bureaucracy. You will find some listed in the resources section for Chapter VI or in the Appendix.

ON FINDING A JOB IN GENERAL

Current Federal Examination Announcements, U.S. Office of Personnel Management. Ask for the recent brochure listing federal job openings, which is available free from your regional or state U.S. Personnel Office (listed in Appendix).

900,000 Plus Jobs Annually; Feingold, S. Norman, and Hansard-Winkler, Glenda Ann. This book presents names and addresses of over 900 trade and professional journals with carry employment want-ads, plus other information for job-seekers. Garrett Park Press, Garrett Park, MD 20896, 1982.

United States Employment Service, now known as Employment Security Offices, a part of the Department of Labor, has offices in most major cities and towns. They are usually combined with state employment services and can be found in the phone book under the government listing for the city or state. For a list of regional offices, see Appendix.

The United States Office of Personnel Management (The Civil Service) has a list of job centers throughout the country. The job center nearest you would be the place to begin your search if you seek federal employment. For a list of regional offices, see Appendix.

For a list of approved employment agencies write the National Employment Association, 2000 K Street, NW, Suite 353, Washington, DC 20036.

FINDING A JOB FOR THE HANDICAPPED

General

Handbook of Selective Placement in Federal Civil Service Employment. U.S. Civil Service Commission, Government Printing Office, Washington, DC 20402. This is an old listing but the most recent. It is free of charge.

Jobs for Handicapped Persons—A New Era in Civil Rights. Public Affairs Pamphlets, 381 Park Avenue South, New York, NY 10016. Distributed by President's Committee on Employment of the Handicapped, 1111 20th Street, NW, Washington, DC 20210.

Jobs for the Disabled. A book by Sar A. Levitan and Robert Taggart, published by Books Demand, UMI.

Jobs Hunting for the Disabled, by Adele Lewis and Edith Marks. Barron, 1983. This book is conclusive and very helpful.

President's Committee on Employment of the Handicapped, address above. This organization promotes maximal employment opportunities for the handicapped and sponsors the annual Employ-the-Handicapped-Week. Write with specific questions or just for general information and listings.

Employment Assistance for the Handicapped. President's Committee on Employment of the Handicapped, address above. This free 37-page pamphlet indicates where to go for guidance and how to find a job, and is an example of the kind of information you can obtain from the President's Committee.

Total Rehabilitation, by George Nelson Wright. Little, Brown and Company, Boston; 1980.

For information on *Sheltered Workshops* in your area, consult your rehabilitation counselor or social worker.

For information on *Day Activity Centers,* check with your local Community Mental Health Center, your rehabilitation counselor, social worker, or the organization that serves persons with your particular handicap.

Specific Handicaps

The best way to obtain employment information on your specific handicap is to write to the organization catering to your needs. Many times they will have listings of job opportunities as well as survey information and specific advice on how to approach potential employers. Listings of these organizations, such as the National Spinal Cord Injury Foundation, the Epilepsy Foundation, the National Multiple Sclerosis

Society, and the Association for Retarded Citizens, to name only a few, can be found in the Appendix. Also, ask the organization if they have any old newsletters that might give you an overview of employment successes or examples of how persons like yourself have obtained jobs.

The other two major sources of information are the President's Committee on the Employment of the Handicapped, which is mentioned several times above, and the U.S. Office of Personnel Management (regional offices are listed in the Appendix). Again, write to them inquiring about employment services related to your specific handicap.

Competitive Employment: New Horizons for Severely Disabled Individuals by Paul Wehman. Paul H. Brooks, Publisher, Baltimore, 1981.

In the Mainstream. 1200 15th Street, NW, Washington, DC 20005. Published six times a year to provide information on affirmative action for the handicapped.

RÉSUMÉS, LETTERS, AND INTERVIEWS

These subjects are covered in the books mentioned in the above section on Finding a Job in General.

The Teenager and the Interview. Richards Rosen Press, 29 East 21st Street, New York, NY 10010.

CHAPTER VI

Your Legal Rights
as a Handicapped Person

Dr. David Hartman began his long campaign to be accepted as a student at a major U.S. medical school while he was still an undergraduate. His father volunteered to help him with the paperwork. They began to fill out the very long and detailed application forms for the schools of his choice. David was a straight-A student in college, yet one by one his applications were rejected. Some schools just sent a routine rejection. Most returned his application fees. A few attempted to explain why he was rejected in spite of his excellent qualifications. It was their judgment that no blind person could ever become a practicing physician. They felt that it was their duty to admit only sighted applicants because the country has such a great need of physicians.

One time just after David had received another rejection, Ralph Nader was visiting the campus, and David had a chance to talk to him. Nader thought legal pressure could be brought against the schools. He suggested that David write a detailed account of his treatment to serve as a starting point for legal action. David was enthusiastic, but when he sat down at his typewriter a voice seemed to caution him. "Wait a minute," it seemed to say. "True, you might force your way into medical school with the help of a court order, but how are the school's administrators going to feel about having their authority challenged? It's going to be tough enough to get through med school. If they are annoyed with you for any reason, they can make it even tougher." He never wrote the letter to Nader. He came to the conclusion that winning a case in court is not the way to win.

Allen Bakke made a different decision. He was admitted to medical school after winning a lawsuit that proved the school had practiced "reverse discrimination" against him.

Our present times have been called "the age of contention" by one American who is dismayed at how avidly we seem to be engaged in suing one another. Potential students sue universities for admission. Husbands sue wives, and wives sue husbands. Roommates sue their roommates. There has been at least one case in which a child sued his parents for not bringing him up right. In the age of contention it is comforting to know that much legislation has been passed to assure the civil rights of handicapped people. But as one handicapped woman put it, "Just when it is our turn to get a piece of the pie, people decided we can no longer afford dessert." Recent budget cuts have caused delays in compliance with the legislation. Nevertheless, it is comforting to know that the law is there to protect you and can be resorted to if needed.

Since 1973 literally thousands of articles and publications have been issued to explain the new legislation and how it applies to the handicapped. The laws are long and complex. They take up hundreds of pages in the Congressional Record. Nowhere have we found a briefer or more concise explanation than that contained in a flyer put out by the Department of Health, Education and Welfare. We reprint it here in its entirety.

A NEW DAY BEGINS FOR DISABLED PERSONS

Are you disabled? Or the parent or guardian of a disabled child? If so, federal law is on your side.

As a physically or mentally disabled person, you have the same right as anyone else to:

- Education
- Employment
- Health care
- Senior citizen activities
- Welfare

and any other public or private service that *U.S. tax dollars help to support.*

If you are otherwise qualified—for a job, college, welfare, or other activity or service—your disability doesn't count. That's the law. It's Title V, section 504, of the Rehabilitation Act of 1973 (Public Law 93–112).

Remember: Your rights are protected by section 504 if your employer, school, college, hospital, or other service provider receives federal assistance. That means federal money, services, or property.

If you're not sure your employer must comply with section 504, ask your supervisor if the activity receives federal assistance. If the answer is "yes," your rights are guaranteed.

If you're not sure your college, hospital, social service agency, or other place that provides services to you must comply with section 504, ask your service representative if the activity receives federal assistance. Again, if the answer is "yes," your rights are guaranteed.

If you are the parent or guardian of a physically or mentally disabled child, you have the right to *demand* that your federally assisted local public school system provide a free education appropriate to your child's needs.

That's the law. In fact, it's two laws: section 504 of the Rehabilitation Act, and the Education for All Handicapped Children Act (Public Law 94–142).

Again, federal assistance is the key. If the public school district in which you live benefits from the use of federal funds, services, or property—and nearly all public school districts do—your disabled child's right to a free appropriate education is assured.

This pamphlet is about your rights under both laws:

- Your section 504 right to work, study, or be served by an institution that receives federal assistance, protected under the Civil Rights Division of the U.S. Department of Justice.
- Your section 504 right to have your disabled child educated at public expense.
- Your right under the Education for All Handicapped Children Act to participate with the public school in planning and evaluating an appropriate learning program for your disabled child.

Is Your Disability Covered?

In the section 504 regulation, a handicapped person is identified as anyone with a physical or mental disability that substantially impairs or restricts one or more of such major life activities as walking, seeing, hearing, speaking, working, or learning. A history of such disability, or the belief on the part of others that a person has such a disability, whether it is so or not, also is recognized as a handicap by the regulation. Handicapping conditions include, but are not limited to:

Alcoholism*

Cancer

---

* The U.S. Attorney General has ruled that alcoholism and drug addiction are physical or mental impairments that are handicapping conditions if they limit one or more of life's major activities.

Cerebral palsy
Deafness or hearing impairment
Diabetes
Drug addiction*
Epilepsy
Heart disease
Mental or emotional illness
Mental retardation
Multiple sclerosis
Muscular dystrophy
Orthopedic, speech, or visual impairment
Perceptual handicaps such as dyslexia, minimal brain dysfunction, developmental aphasia.

Your Right to Employment

As a disabled job applicant or employee, you have the same rights and benefits as nonhandicapped applicants and employees.

Your ability, training, and experience must be considered. Your disability must *not* be considered—unless it keeps you from doing the job adequately.

An employer receiving federal assistance may not discriminate against you in:

• Recruitment, advertising, or processing of applications for employment.

You can't be required to take a physical examination before a job is offered. You may be required to take a physical examination after the job is offered if the examination is required of other applicants.

This provision is to prevent discrimination against persons with such hidden disabilities as heart disease and epilepsy that would be revealed in a physical examination. It is also to keep employers from requiring a physical examination for handicapped job applicants only—a common practice in the past—then denying them a job because they failed to pass the examination.

• Hiring, promotion or demotion, transfer, layoff, or rehiring.
• Job assignments or career ladders.
• Leaves of absence, sick leave, training programs, and other fringe benefits.

Once hired, your employer is required to take reasonable steps to accommodate your disability unless they would cause the employer undue hardship. That may mean supplying, for example:

- A reader if you are blind and the job includes paperwork.
- An interpreter if you are deaf and the job requires telephone contacts.
- Adequate workspace and access to it if you use a wheelchair.
- Minor adjustment in working hours if you are required to visit a methadone clinic daily.

Your Right to Health Care

Hospitals are the largest group of health care providers affected by the section 504 regulation.

As a disabled person, you are entitled to all medical services and medically related instruction available to the public. Hospitals receiving federal assistance (including Medicare payments) must take steps to accommodate your disability.

Among other things, hospitals must:

- Provide an emergency room interpreter or make other effective provisions for deaf patients.
- Treat the physical injury of a person under the influence of alcohol or drugs.
- Admit disabled persons to natural childbirth, antismoking, and other public-service programs of instruction.

Federally assisted long-term health care facilities may:
Operate separate programs for different physical disabilities and mental disorders.

For example, a sanitarium for patients with lung disease is *not* required to have a mental health program for a patient with lung disease and an emotional disorder.

On the other hand, the institution may not exclude a person with lung disease who also has other handicaps.

If your disabled child is in a long-term health care facility:
The facility and the local public school district are jointly responsible for providing a free appropriate education for your child.

If you are a Medicaid patient, your private physician must:

- Have an office physically accessible to you,
- Treat you in a hospital or your home, or, if this is not possible,

- Refer you to another physician whose office is accessible, after conferring with you.

Services provided to you as a Medicare patient in a federally assisted hospital *are* covered under section 504; services provided by a private physician *are not.*

Your Right to Social and Rehabilitation Services

As a disabled person, you have the right to participate in vocational rehabilitation, senior citizen activities, day care (for your disabled child), or any other social service program receiving federal assistance on an equal basis with nonhandicapped persons.

For example, you *may not:*

- Be denied admission because you use a wheelchair and need access to classrooms, recreation areas, or buses.
- Be excluded from vocational training because you are blind, mentally retarded, or paralyzed and may need more training for paid employment than students with other disabilities.

Your Right to Education

As a disabled young person or adult, you have the same right as anyone else to go to college or enroll in a job training or adult post-high school basic education program.

The college, job-training, or adult basic education program you select must consider your application on the basis of your academic and other school records. Your disability is not a factor.

A college or training program *may not,* for example:

- Ask you to take a pre-admission test that inadequately measures your academic level because no special provisions were made for the fact that you are blind, deaf, or otherwise disabled.
- Inquire about any disability before admitting you, unless it is trying to overcome the effects of prior limitations on enrollment of handicapped students, and you are willing to volunteer the information.
- Limit the number of handicapped students admitted.

Colleges are *not* required to lower academic standards or alter degree requirements for you.

But, depending on your disability, they *may* have to:

- Extend the time allowed for you to earn a degree or substitute one elective course for another.
- Modify teaching methods and examinations so you can fully participate in a degree program.
- Provide braille books or other aids for you if they are not available from other sources.

These section 504 protections apply to all public and private education institutions receiving assistance.

Your Disabled Child's Right to Education

No later than school year 1978–79, your state and local school district must provide under section 504 an appropriate elementary and secondary education for your physically or mentally disabled child. This public education must cost you no more than it costs parents of nonhandicapped children.

This is true no matter which of the following education settings you and your public school district decide is best for your child.

- A regular public school classroom.
- A special education public school program.
- A residential school if the public school has no appropriate program.
- An appropriate education in a hospital if your child is receiving long-term patient care.

Your public school district *must* provide an education for your child regardless of the type or severity of his or her disability.

You and your child have even more specific protection under the Education for All Handicapped Children Act.

The Act says your state *must:*

- Locate every disabled child and young person, age 6–17, living in the state by September 1, 1978 and begin their education at public expense.
- If public education is required for children age 3–5, locate them by September 1, 1978 and begin their education at public expense.
- If public education is required for disabled youth, age 18–21, locate them by September 1, 1980 and begin an appropriate program for them at public expense.
- Give priority attention, first, to disabled children receiving no public education and, second, to the most severely handicapped children

in each disability group who are currently receiving an inadequate education.

The Education for All Handicapped Children Act says you and your public school district should work together in the interest of your child's education, happiness, and physical and emotional well-being.

The school district must develop—with your advice and consent—an individualized education program for your child and give you *in writing:*

- A statement of learning goals it will try to help your child reach.
- A list of special aids which will be provided such as braille books if your child is blind or a high desk if your child uses a wheelchair.
- A schedule to review periodically your child's progress and, with your consent, make program revisions as needed.
- An explanation of your rights of due process under the law which include your right to written notice from the school of major changes proposed in your child's program or program location.

What You Can Do

If you feel that your rights have been violated by a business, hospital, physician, school, college, or any other institution receiving HEW assistance, because of your disability or your child's disability, write, giving details to:

Office for Civil Rights, Department of Education in *your* region, whose address is listed below.

Region I (Conn., Maine, Mass., N.H., R.I., Vt.)
J.W. McCormick Post Office and Court House
Boston, MA 02109

Region II (N.J., N.Y., Puerto Rico, Virgin Isles)
26 Federal Plaza—33rd Floor
New York, N.Y. 10278

Region III (Del., D.C., Md., Pa., Va., W. Va.)
3535 Market Street
Philadelphia, PA 19104

Region IV (Ala., Fla., Ga., Ky., Miss., N.C., S.C., Tenn.)
101 Marietta Street, NW
Atlanta, Ga. 30323

Region V (Ill., Ind., Mich., Minn., Ohio, Wis.)
300 South Wacker Drive
Chicago, Ill. 60606

Region VI (Ark., La., N.M., Okla., Texas)
1200 Main Tower Bldg.
Dallas, Texas 75202

Region VII (Iowa, Kan., Mo., Neb.)
324 East 11th Street
Kansas City, Mo. 64106

Region VIII (Colo., Mont., N.D., S.D., Utah, Wyo.)
Federal Bldg.
1961 Stout St.
Denver, Colo. 80294

Region IX (Ariz., Calif., Hawaii, Nev., Guam, Trust Terr. Pac.
Isles, Amer. Samoa)
1275 Market Street, 14th Floor
San Francisco, CA 94103

Region X (Alaska, Idaho, Ore., Wash.)
2901 Third Avenue, M/S106
Seattle Wash. 98101

The Office for Civil Rights enforces federal laws prohibiting discrimination against persons on the basis of race, color, national origin, religion, sex, age, or mental and physical handicap and investigates discrimination complaints brought by individuals under these statutes.

Civil Rights Division
U.S. Department of Justice
Federal Enforcement Office, Room 4712
Tenth and Constitution Avenues, NW
Washington, DC 20530

Other Rights

In addition to your section 504 rights discussed above, Title V of the Rehabilitation Act and the Developmental Disability Act give you other equal opportunity protections.

You have the right to be considered for federal employment.

Section 501 requires that federal agencies take affirmative action to hire and promote disabled persons.

All executive branch agencies must make an annual report to the Civil Service Commission on their progress in hiring and promoting disabled persons. The Civil Service Commission in turn reports to Congress.

If you believe you have been denied a federal job because of your handicap, contact the Federal Job Information Center nearest you. Consult your local telephone directory for the address and telephone number.

If you believe you have been denied a promotion in a federal agency because of your handicap, contact the Equal Employment Opportunity Officer in your agency.

You have the right of access to federal and federally financed buildings.

Section 502 sets up a federal compliance board to make sure disabled persons have access to all buildings owned, occupied, or financed by the U.S. government.

If you have a complaint about an inaccessible building, write, giving details to:

> Architectural and Transportation Barriers Compliance Board
> Mary E. Switzer Building, Room 1010
> 330 C Street, SW
> Washington, DC 20202

You have the right to be considered for employment or service by federal contractors.

Section 503 says firms doing business with the U.S. government must take affirmative action to hire and promote disabled persons.

If you believe your rights have been violated, file a complaint within 120 days of the alleged violation with:

> Veterans and Handicapped Division,
> Office of Federal Contract Compliance
> Programs, Department of Labor
> Washington, D.C. 20210

Rights of persons with developmental disabilities:

The Developmental Disability Services and Facilities Construction Act, as amended, protects you:

If you are mentally retarded or have cerebral palsy, epilepsy, or autism—or dyslexia resulting from these conditions—you are entitled to state legal protection and expanded services effective October 1977. States were required by this date to have a system in place to investigate your complaint and take appropriate legal or administrative action.

If you have a complaint, write:

Administration on Developmental Disabilities
Department of Education
Washington, DC 20201

Information About Federal Programs

For information about specific programs serving disabled persons, write to the appropriate federal agency listed below.

Health Care Financing Administration
200 Independence Avenue, SW
Washington, DC 20201

Administers Medicare and Medicaid and sets standards for the quality of health care under these programs.

Office of Information and Resources for the Handicapped
U.S. Department of Education
Mary E. Switzer Building, Room 3119
330 C Street, SW
Washington, DC 20202

Gives assistance to states and local school districts to improve their services to handicapped students; to research efforts and demonstration projects which encourage innovation and improve programs; to education institutions to aid staff members and volunteers training in special education; and to the general public and specific populations through public media, captioned films, and Closer Look, the National Information Center for the Handicapped.

Office of Human Developmental Services
Department of Health and Human Services
Washington, DC 20201

Administers Head Start and other child development services, vocational and other rehabilitation programs of the Rehabilitation Services Administration, programs to assist persons with developmental disabilities, and programs for older Americans; also family counseling, child welfare, and related social services.

Public Health Service
200 Independence Avenue, SW
Washington, DC 20201

Administers maternal and child health, family planning, and services to disabled children; also research, staff training, and service grants under the Alcohol, Drug Abuse, and Mental Health Administration to improve alcohol, drug abuse, and mental health care; and a variety of disabling disease research activities under the National Institutes of Health.

Social Security Administration
6401 Security Building
Baltimore, MD 21235

Administers retirement, survivors and disability insurance benefits; supplemental security income for aged, blind, and disabled persons; and aid to families with dependent children.

If you would like general information on obtaining and protecting your rights to education, housing, employment, transportation, or health care, write:

American Coalition of Citizens with Disabilities
1200 Fifteenth Street, NW, Suite 201
Washington, DC 20005

CONCLUSION

As you can see from the preceding "brief" summary, obtaining your rights or even just understanding what they are is not easy. Fortunately most government and private agencies that serve the handicapped have legal experts who will help you with any problem that may arise. Many publish legal newsletters that may be available to you. Other suggestions on how to find help if you should need it are in the resources section.

Be sure you have thought it over very carefully before you resort to using lawyers and the courts to achieve your rights. Consider some of the following:

1. How important is it to me and to my future to prove this point in court?
2. Can I afford the amount of time and unpleasantness it may involve?
3. Can I afford the legal fees and court costs?
4. Can I locate any other sources of financial assistance?

5. Am I running any risk of winning the battle but losing the war? By this we mean that it would mean little to achieve a job through a court order if the suit had stirred up so much bitterness on both sides that working there would be extremely unpleasant.

Your legal rights apply to every aspect of your life. To name just a few: they apply to your school life, your work and career life, your personal life, your recreational life, your life as a citizen of your country, your state, and your home town. Understanding your rights and how to go about gaining redress when they have been violated can add much to your general satisfaction in life.

In the remaining chapters we shall consider some of the elements that make up the life-styles of nearly everybody and discuss some of the options open to you as an adult member of the community of the handicapped.

SELECTED RESOURCES CHAPTER VI— YOUR LEGAL RIGHTS

Notes: Some listed publications are free, some cost a little, and some are expensive. Ask the price or include a line saying "Send only if it costs less than $1.00 or $5.00" or whatever.

CIVIL RIGHTS IN GENERAL

Organizations

Equal Employment Opportunities Commission, Office of Public Affairs, 2401 E Street, NW, Washington, DC 20506

Office of Civil Rights, U.S. Department of Health, Personnel Office, Washington, DC 20201.

League of Women Voters, Publications Department, 1730 M Street, NW, Washington, DC 20036.

Publications

Know Your Civil Rights: What You Should Know About Equal Employment Opportunity, published by E.E.O.C., address above.

Going to Court in the Public Interest, League of Women Voters, address above, or call a local chapter office.

The Verdict Is In: A Look at Public Interest Litigation, League of Women Voters, address above, or call a local chapter office.

CIVIL RIGHTS OF THE HANDICAPPED

Organizations

Note: Most of the following organizations have legal divisions and put out numerous publications. Most also offer information and referral services. Some offer direct assistance. Be sure your request is specific when you write.

American Coalition of Citizens with Disabilities, 1200 15th Street, NW, Suite 201, Washington, DC 20005.

Disability Rights Center, Inc., 1345 Connecticut Avenue, Suite 1124, Washington, DC 20036.

Regional Rehabilitation Research Institute on Attitudinal, Legal and Leisure Barriers, 1828 L Street, NW, Suite 704, Washington, DC 20036.

Council for Exceptional Children, 1920 Associations Drive, Reston, VA 22091.

Mental Health Law Project, 12219 19th Street, NW, Washington, DC 20036.

Mental Disability Legal Resource Center, American Bar Association, Commission on the Mentally Disabled, 1800 M Street, NW, Washington, DC 20036.

The National Center for Law and the Deaf, Gallaudet College, Florida Avenue and Seventh Street, NE, Washington, DC 20002.

Division of the Blind and Physically Handicapped, U.S. Library of Congress, Washington, DC 20540.

Publications

Affirmative Action for Disabled People—A Pocket Guide. President's Committee on Employment of the Handicapped, Government Printing Office, Washington, DC 20402.

Handbook on Employment Rights of the Handicapped, by S. Herrman and L. Walker. George Washington University, Regional Rehabilitation Institute, Washington, DC., 1978.

A Handbook on the Legal Rights of Handicapped People, President's Committee on Employment of the Handicapped, Washington, DC 20210. This 103-page handbook covers your rights to benefits, education, employment, hospital services, housing, and transportation and lists lawyers and organizations that can be of service.

The Handicapping of America, by Frank Bowe. A book on barriers and legal rights, published by the American Coalition of Citizens with Handicaps, 1200 15th Street, NW, Suite 201, Washington, DC 20005

Know Your Rights: The Disabled Voter's Guide, 1984 Edition. American Foundation for the Blind, 15 West 16th Street, New York, NY 10011.

Overdue Process: Providing Legal Services to Disabled Clients. Regional Rehabilitation Research Institute on Attitudinal, Legal and Leisure Barriers, 1828 L Street, NW, Suite 704, Washington, DC 20036. Twenty-four pages.

Reprints of Public Law 94–42 or Education for All Handicapped Children Act of 1975, and The 503 and 504 Legislation of the Rehabilitation Act of 1973. Office of Alumnae Public Relations, Gallaudet Alumnae Newsletter.

The Rights of Mentally Retarded Persons: An American Civil Liberties Handbook, by Paul R. Friedman. Avon, 1976.

There Oughta Be a Law—There Is. A series of pamphlets covering employment discrimination, job accommodation, accessibility, and affirmative action. Mainstream Inc., 1200 15th Street, NW, Washington, DC 20005.

Word From Washington. A newsletter of the United Cerebral Palsy Association, Inc., 66 East 34th Street, New York, NY 10016.

TELEPHONE ASSISTANCE

Mainstream Legislative Hotline. Mainstream, Inc., a nonprofit organization that promotes the mainstreaming of disabled people in employment and education, recently added a TTY communication unit and a toll-free WATS line. You may call for information on your rights or on many other aspects of daily living and working.

Office for Civil Rights has recently installed special equipment on which deaf persons can send and receive typed messages through standard telephone lines. The list of regional offices, the numbers that can be called by teletypewriter, and the states served by each regional office follow:

Boston   617-223-1111
(Connecticut, Maine, Massachusetts, New Hampshire, Rhode Island, Vermont)

New York   212–264-9464
(New Jersey, New York, Puerto Rico, Virgin Islands)

Philadelphia   215-596-6794
(Delaware, D.C., Maryland, Pennsylvania, Virginia, West Virginia)

Atlanta   404-221-2010
(Alabama, Florida, Georgia, Kentucky, Mississippi, North Carolina, South Carolina, Tennessee)

Chicago   312-353-2540
(Illinois, Indiana, Minnesota, Michigan, Ohio, Wisconsin)

Dallas   214-767-3983
(Arkansas, Louisiana, New Mexico, Oklahoma, Texas)

Kansas City   816-374-7264
(Iowa, Kansas, Missouri, Nebraska)

Denver   303-844-3417
(Colorado, Montana, North Dakota, South Dakota, Utah, Wyoming)

San Francisco   415-227-8124
(Arizona, California, Hawaii, Nevada, Guam, American Samoa)

Seattle   206-442-4542
(Alaska, Idaho, Oregon, Washington)

Headquarters   202-732-1467
(Washington, D.C.)

CHAPTER VII

Your Life-style—
Can It Be Planned?

"Independent living is a new concept in the rehabilitation of handicapped people. Its driving principle is to provide services to severely handicapped individuals which will enable them to become fully functional members of society."

"The essence of independent living is control over one's life. The concept focuses upon the individual's ability to choose and achieve a desired life-style."

The above two quotations are from Chapter III of a 1978 report to the President by the National Health Care Policies for the Handicapped Working Group of the President's Committee on Employment of the Handicapped.

When *Roger Meyers* was growing up in the 1950's, the only future for a retarded person seemed to be in an institution for the retarded. The only life-style available was an "institutional" one. Roger's family rejected this path. Ultimately he became a beneficiary of the new U.S. policy of treating handicapped people as much as possible like everyone else and of providing the kind of assistance for them that permits them to grow and develop their full potentials. Roger and his wife, Virginia, now live in their own apartment. With their Supplementary Security incomes, plus what Roger earns at his full-time job as a busboy, they are living, as the title of the book about them suggests, *Like Normal People.*[1]

"Life-style" is one of those popular words that have only recently found their way into dictionaries. Style is a manner of doing something. Life-style means the manner of doing just about everything in your

---

[1] Meyers, Robert. *Like Normal People.* McGraw-Hill Book Co., New York, NY, 1978.

life whether it relates to your work life, your recreational life, or your private life.

When you are a child your life-style is a part of your family's. This usually seems entirely right to you. As a teenager you are probably discovering that there are some aspects of your parents' life-style that you would change if you had anything to say about it. These first stirrings of your personal preferences are the beginning of your own adult life-style.

Can a life-style really be planned? The answer to this question is yes and no. Probably you will never achieve the detail and precision in planning your life-style that is often possible in planning for a career. But if you give enough careful thought to your life-style, you can move toward it just as you can move toward a satisfactory career.

HOW TO BUILD A LIFE-STYLE

You can build a richly rewarding life-style for yourself if you give careful thought to the following three aspects. First, define and learn to recognize and understand your preferences in a very broad range of areas. Second, plan your life-style to fit within your expected budget. And third, accept and build around any "givens" with which life and your handicap present you.

Define Your Preferences

Reviewing some of the lists you have made earlier will get you started on this analysis. If you have taken any interest inventory tests they may yield some valuable insights. To get you started we suggest just a few questions you might answer in three of the major areas.

Human relationships: What types of relationships with others do I enjoy? To what groups do I belong? Or would like to belong? Church, temple, synagogue? Fraternal organization? Hobby group? Bridge or other social club? Political action group? Or what? List your preferences.

Housing and living arrangements: What kind of housing do I prefer? Apartment? House? Group home? Mobile home? Do I prefer to live alone or with others? In the city, suburbs, or country? In what part of the country?

Recreational preferences: Active participation. Sports? Which ones? Photography? Amateur theater? Amateur painting? Singing or choral groups? Pottery-making? Other crafts? Playing a musical instrument? Participating in a dance or other hobby group? *Spectator activities.* Spectator sports? Which ones? Museums? Exhibits? Attending theaters? Movies? Concerts? Ballets? Other? *Collecting.* Stamps? Coins? Antiques? Other?

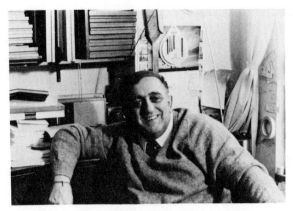

Fred Mancuso

Your Life-style and Your Budget

The following exchange was overheard on a bus. "George really knows how to live! Last Friday he caught an overnight flight to London. He saw a show and went to a party on Saturday and flew home on Sunday."

"I guess that really qualifies him for membership in the jet set," his companion replied, "that and his batching it in a three-bedroom apartment in Manhattan."

It is true that the rich and super-rich usually have grander and more money-oriented life-styles. Yet not all wealthy people adopt the jet-set way of life. Every now and then one reads a story in the paper of a poor old woman or man who had been living in a shack at the edge of the town dump. Usually he or she received welfare and an occasional visit from a social worker. One day the social worker found the client dead. When the premises were searched, thousands of dollars were found stashed away in a gunnysack or stuffed in a lumpy mattress. The moral of the story is that you can live with a more humble life-style than your income would support or any life-style within your means.

By deciding on a career area, you have already made the principal decision about how much money in general you will have to support your life-style. If the occupation you have chosen doesn't seem to pay enough to support your ideal life-style, some compromises may need to be made. Before you compromise in favor of earning more money, however, remember some good advice from *Fred Mancuso,* the Canadian artist you met in Chapter III. "No matter how small the wage may be, the one advice I can give you—as long as you are happy doing whatever you are doing—this is the secret of being a success." Being happy on a year-round basis is more important to Fred, and to most of us, than having more money to spend in expensive recreations.

Accept Your "Givens"

Every person ever born was born into a set of circumstances or "givens" over which he or she has little or no control. "I didn't ask to be born," some dissatisfied young people and adults are heard to wail. That is the reason they give for rejecting everything or anything about the society in which they live. They *didn't* ask to be born, but then, neither did anyone else.

It has occurred to nearly everyone while passing through periods of rebellion that "If I could have selected my parents, I would have made a better choice!" Parents are the first and most obvious of every person's givens. The shape and general condition of our bodies are also givens. Some are destined to be short, some tall. Some are men, some women. Some are handicapped, some are physically almost perfect. Most are somewhere in between. Our givens are the boundaries within which we must operate. They are the framework around which we must construct our lives.

One of the authors worked at a preschool for severely handicapped children. The children were often brought in after their parents had been told by doctors or other professionals that "Your child will never walk," or "Your child's intelligence is too low for him to attend public school," or "Because of the neuromuscular involvement your child may never learn to talk." It didn't always happen, of course, but time after time these givens pronounced on very young children proved not to be true. They were overcome, or partially overcome, by the determination and hard work of the children themselves and of those who worked with them.

Perhaps you have already overcome certain childhood givens.

You may have developed a way of working with and around your givens to your own best advantage. A now forgotten oriental philosopher worked out the best way of handling givens. His words are so workable that many people keep them framed where they will be reminded of them often:

God grant me the *strength* to accept the things I cannot change,
the *courage* to change the things I can change, and,
the *wisdom* to know the difference.

Victoria Conley is a rehabilitation counselor in Alton, Illinois. A quadraplegic who drives her own converted van, she was disabled by a crippling disease from the age of six. She says, "The fact that I am a woman and disabled is obvious and irrefutable. But these are only labels and tell only a partial story. I am me and comprised of many labels: single, counselor, driver, daughter, sister, friend, peer, feminist, shy, assertive, educated, woman, and disabled. And this is only a partial list." Victoria is building a successful career and life-style around her givens.[2]

Some of the toughest problems imaginable in accepting one's givens are presented to an increasing number of young people who are becoming crippled in their teens through automobile, motorcycle, or sporting accidents. The mother of *Gene Williams,* whom you met in Chapter III, summed up this traumatic experience. "It's like a death in the family. You mourn for what you've lost, but you know you've got to go on. So you gradually accept it and you do whatever you can do."

Joni Eareckson (Chapter III), paralyzed by a diving accident when she was in high school, described what she went through in accepting her new set of givens. "I recalled hearing a preacher say one time that God never closes a door but that he opens a window. I took the promise at face value and waited. And as I waited I began to come to grips with myself. There were some things that were not going to happen. I would never walk. I probably would never marry, but there were some other things I could do. Some options were left. I began to lay out my future, lining up the positive things I had on my side of the ledger. I quit questioning God about the whys of my life and began asking Him how."[3]

HOW MUCH CAN TECHNOLOGY HELP YOU?

In Chapter VI you read about *Orlo Nichols,* actuary who works for the Social Security Administration in Baltimore. He makes use of an amazing array of aids to communication. These range from the familiar telephone, typewriter, and dictating machine to a braille calculator, a keypunch machine, and an opticon. An opticon, or Optical to Tactile Converter, is a small three- or four-pound instrument that looks like a tape recorder. It has a miniature attachment that looks something like a microphone. Actually, it is a tiny electric-eye camera. The camera scans a page of print and sends a signal to the machine. The signal activates a system of vibrating pins on a flat panel. The pins form

[2] *Rehabilitation Gazette 77.*
[3] Erickson, Joni. "There's Only One Handicap in Life." *Guideposts,* July 1977, p. 6.

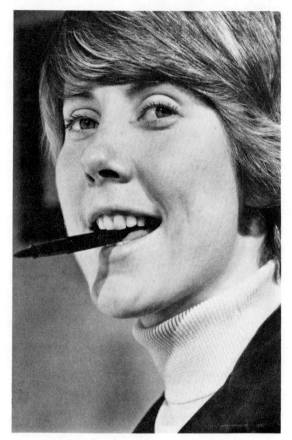

Joni Eareckson holds a drawing pen.

raised letters and numbers identical to the material on the page being scanned. Although it does not translate the message into the braille alphabet, the blind user can read the raised letters in the same way he reads braille. The equipment Orlo uses represents only a small percentage of the many ways that have been or are now being worked out for blind persons. They can now function in a world that depends heavily on sight to transmit its communications.

For the deaf there are also many new helpful devices. Telephones that can be used by the deaf are already in service at eleven regional offices and headquarters of the Office for Civil Rights of the U.S. Department of Health, Education and Welfare. Flashing lights serve as doorbells and alarm clocks for the deaf. More and more "hearing dogs" are being trained to alert their deaf masters that someone is at the door.

There is an ever-growing variety of imaginative devices to assist partially paralyzed people to do everything from hoisting themselves in and out of bed to typewriting, eating, and dressing. The invention some years ago of the electric wheelchair made mobility possible for many more severely handicapped persons. Prototype models of wheelchairs that climb stairs are now being used.

No matter what kind of disability you have, you will want to keep abreast of all the latest technological advances. Be sure you are availing yourself of any that would be of particular help. You will find some selected references to sources at the end of this chapter. Some references to periodicals that serve as a means of keeping up to date will be found at the end of Chapter X.

INDEPENDENT LIVING—THE STATE OF THE ART

New Patterns for the Young

The popular life-style among most American young people is to move out of their parents' home and establish independent living quarters. Most do this when they get their first full-time job. Others, with their parents' consent, do it even earlier. Independent living from the earliest possible age seems to be the way to go. Many who do this, however, are in for a kind of cultural shock. Many things just seem to happen in the homes in which they grew up. Now for the first time they find they have to figure out a way to do everything for themselves. No one brews a pot of coffee and has it ready on the stove so you can help yourself before you go to work. There's no one to wake you in time if you happen to sleep through your alarm. There is no special day when you can put out things to go to the cleaner. No one washes your clothes unless you lug a load off to the laundromat. No one cleans up the house. When you come home from work, the bed you left unmade and the dishes you left in the sink will be just as you left them. When you receive a package you have to track it down at the Post Office on the following Saturday, because no one is at home to receive it. You have to think about meals and cooking. You have to buy the food and remember to pay the rent and telephone bills. Toughest of all, you have to do all this and more without spending more money than you earn.

Independent living for young people is a life-style that has developed rather recently. In the eighteenth and early nineteenth centuries we were an agricultural society. Young people continued to live at home and work on the family farm until they married and set up homes of their own. When people moved increasingly to the cities, it still was usual for the young people to live with their families even when they had obtained jobs in factories, offices, or stores. Now, independent living as the new life-style for the young is being made possible also for handicapped people.

Much remains to be analyzed and understood before a maximum number of handicapped persons may be mainstreamed into independent living. New skills need to be learned by many handicapped persons themselves. Progress is being made toward finding alternatives for living in institutions, in at least three areas:

Needs of the handicapped are being studied. The physical and social needs of handicapped persons as they relate to the larger communities into which they will be moved are being studied. The daily living skills they will need are being evaluated. Courses in rehabilitation for daily life activities are being developed and taught.

Independent living quarters. As the new federal programs get under way, it now appears there will be at least two alternatives to living in an institution. One is to set up the handicapped person in independent living quarters and provide for him or her any necessary services and attendants. These persons can usually work full or part time although they may still need special services and more income than they can earn. They are assisted by the federal program of Supplementary Security Income.

Group homes. Not all handicapped persons want to live alone. Some are not capable of doing so. In several parts of the country large houses have been redesigned to be barrier-free. A number of handicapped persons live in such a home and share the needed attendants and other service personnel. Each person has his or her own quarters. Residents can go to and come from work or social engagements as they would from any other home.

A POSSIBLE STUMBLING BLOCK

There is one possible barrier to the development of your life-style of which you should be aware. The barrier is posed by the tangle of rules and regulations that provide for the handicapped. Several aspects of the problem are illustrated by the story of *Cass Irvine* of Louisville, Kentucky, which appeared in *Rehabilitation Gazette 77.* She is a polio quad since the age of nine. Here, in her own words, is her story.

"I graduated from college in 1968 with a BA in English. In 1973

I moved from my parents' home into an apartment of my own with a companion-attendant. I received my MA in English in 1974 and began my present work as a part-time instructor of English at Jefferson Community College.

"During the summer of 1975, my radicalization started to happen. I began to realize that no matter how hard I worked, I could never work hard enough to become economically self-sufficient. I do not have the physical stamina to work enough hours to totally support myself and related expenses (i.e., companion, special transportation, equipment, etc.). My family will always have to pay many of my bills, and they are trying to provide financial security for me after they are gone.

"This all began to anger me. This and the realization that it took so long to find a companion—my only solution to independent living. (How odd to depend one's entire life on another and call it independence!)

"I was lucky enough to find an older apartment that is accessible and a companion who is congenial. Once settled into my financial (thanks to my family) and socially (thanks to me!) independent life, I decided to look for alternative financial aids. My luck began to backfire. I found that I did not make enough money teaching part time to support my expenses, but I made too much while working to receive any aid. If I did not work, I still would not receive enough aid to pay my expenses. But what I did find out was that I could receive enough money to live in an institution."

With the new policy of moving persons out of institutions and into independent living arrangements, only the most severely handicapped will remain in institutions. However, there have been many reports of handicapped persons living independently and working who have had to quit working because their salaries were too large to qualify them for Supplementary Security Income or other special services they could not live without. Yet their salaries were not large enough to cover all these extra expenses on their own. Inflation is making this problem even worse. Hopefully, such regulations, which deny many handicapped persons the privilege of making whatever contribution they can make to the world, will be adjusted to remove this disincentive to work.

DECISIONS YOU CAN PUT OFF

There are great events in most people's lives that have a big effect on life-style. One such event is finding the appropriate person to marry. Many of the people you have met earlier in this book are happily married. Some are married to other handicapped persons, some to nonhandi-

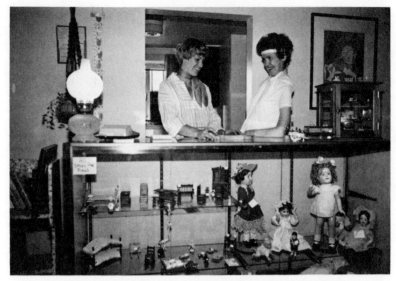

Mary Ann Hamilton, with her daughter, Mrs. Pat Jenni (left).

capped persons. Many are raising children. The patterns are as varied as the persons themselves.

Then there are many strong marriages that have survived the trauma of having one of the partners crippled by disease or accident. *Mary Ann Hamilton* of Denver, Colorado, became a respiratory polio quad more than twenty-five years ago. At the time she had been married only a few years and had four small children. Now that her children are grown, she says, "As I look back from this pinnacle of survival, I see that my husband, my children, and I have maneuvered through an era of turmoil that destroyed many families. Perhaps we survived and flourished because my polio was a buffer, an object of intense concern that served as an adhesive to hold our family together, keeping our idea of what is important, simple."[4]

For many years rehabilitation agencies have considered homemaking to be a career. They offer guidance and training in homemaking skills that are useful to handicapped men or women living alone as well as to handicapped wives.

Rehabilitation counselors are increasingly being trained for counseling on the most intimate aspects of sex and family life. Some ways of finding this kind of advice are listed in the resources section.

---

[1] *Rehabilitation Gazette 77,* p. 8.

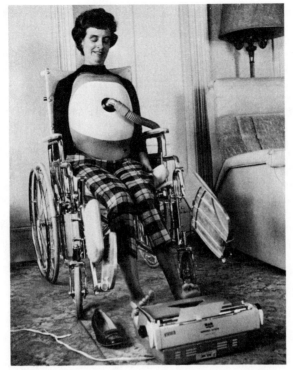

Donna McGuinn, a successful writer in spite of everything.

CONCLUSION

The new legislation makes it possible for many more handicapped people to develop life-styles that satisfy them. But the primary responsibility for developing a satisfying life-style rests with you. There have always been handicapped persons who managed to develop a positive life-style in spite of everything. One such person was *Donna McGwinn.* Donna was a polio quad who was totally dependent upon a respirator and an aspirator. For many years she was a successful writer. She lived alone with one live-in attendant. She was in complete control of her life. The following quote is taken from a tribute written at the time of her death in 1978 in a magazine where her articles frequently appeared.[5] "She managed her household and her attendant with dignity and efficiency. She was always immaculately and smartly groomed.

---

[5] *Rehabilitation Gazette* 77, p. 1.

She had a charming home. She entertained graciously. She had a wealth of friends. She loved. She was loved. She lived a full, independent and productive life."

Donna was just sixteen years old when polio struck her down. That is about the same age that *Gene Williams* was when he met with a high school wrestling accident that turned him into a quadraplegic. Since then he has met all the challenges confronting a person who is being rehabilitated for wheelchair living. He seems to have resolved to do as much as possible with his life. So far he has served as media director in a political campaign, a job that called for him to drive more than 35,000 miles. He has attended Harvard where he studied musicology, political science, psychology, somatic medicine, and neuroanatomy. He has made two trips to Mexico completely on his own. As he puts it, "I was tossing myself up for grabs." He just wanted to prove how much he could do. He also became a jazz percussionist with his own progressive jazz group. This was taken from a 1973 report. We don't know what Gene is doing now, but one thing is sure. He is living the kind of life he wants to lead and he is making a unique contribution to the world around him.

SELECTED RESOURCES CHAPTER VII—LIFE-STYLE

Notes: Information has been listed in this section in the order the subjects were discussed earlier in the chapter.

Some listed publications are free, some cost a little, and some are expensive. Ask the price, or include a line saying "Send only if it costs less than $1.00 or $5.00" or whatever.

* indicates books that can usually be found in public libraries or in your guidance or rehabilitation counselor's office.

TECHNOLOGICAL AIDS TO LIFE-STYLE

Disability and Rehabilitation Handbook. Robert M. Goldenson et al. McGraw-Hill, 1978. Source book for addresses for all kinds of aids useful at work and at home.

Educational Materials Catalog. Sister Kenny Institute, 800 East 28th Street at Chicago Avenue, Minneapolis, MN 55407. The Sister Kenney Institute is a valuable source of information. It investigates, promotes, and supports rehabilitation projects, specializes in treatment of acute or chronic disabled persons, and offers professional educational programs in the most recent rehabilitation practices.

Ideas for Better Living. A catalogue published by the American Foundation for the Blind, 15 West 16th Street, New York, NY 10011.

The Kurzweil Report: Technology for the Handicapped. A promotional newsletter published by the Kurzweil Computer Products Co., 185 Albany Street, Cambridge, MA 02139.

Library of Congress, Reference Service. National Library Service for the Blind and Physically Handicapped, Library of Congress, 1291 Taylor Street, NW, Washington, DC 20542. Ask for information relating to reading, writing, and other communications for the visually and physically handicapped person.

National Homecaring Council, 253 Park Avenue South, New York, NY 10003. Ask for the *Directory of Accredited/Approved Homemaker-Home Health Aide Services,* an annual publication.

Telephone add-ons. Contact any telephone company business office. The Bell Telephone Systems booklet on services for special needs describes modifications available upon request.

INDEPENDENT LIVING—HOMEMAKING—FAMILY LIFE

General

Accent on Living Buyer's Guide, 1984-1985: Your Number One Source of Information on Products for the Disabled, 4th ed. Betty Garee, Cheever Publications. This 128-page guide lists names and addresses of manufacturers of products for the disabled. $10.00 in paperback.

Disabled? Yes. Defeated? No, by Kathleen Cruzic. Spectrum Books, 1982. Prentice-Hall, Inc., Englewood Cliffs, N.J. 07632. This complete book covers all aspects of living.

Independent Living for the Handicapped and Elderly, by Elizabeth E. May, Neva Waggoner, and Eleanor Hotte. Houghton Mifflin, Boston MA 02107.

Living Fully, by Sol Gordon. Ed-U Press, 760 Ostrum Avenue, Syracuse, NY 13210. A guide for young people with handicaps.

No Place Like Home—Alternative Living Arrangements for Teenagers and Adults with Cerebral Palsy. United Cerebral Palsy Association, 66 East 34th Street, New York, NY 10016.

The Right to Choose, Achieving Residential Alternatives in the Community. National Association for Retarded Citizens, 2709 Avenue E East, Arlington, TX 76011.

The Source Book for the Disabled, by Glorya Hale. HR and W, 1982.

What You Can Do for Yourself, by Patricia Galbraith. Drake Publishers, Inc., New York, NY. A wheelchairer writes about daily living aids.

Other

Accent on Living, Special Publications, Box 700, Bloomington, IL 61701. The Disabled Person and Family Dynamics, Sexuality and the Disabled Female, Sex and the Spinal Cord Injured.

Adaptations and Techniques for the Disabled Homemaker. Sister Kenny Institute (address above).

Clothing Designs for the Handicapped, Anne Kernalequen. Accent Special Publications (address above).

The Hidden Minority: America's Handicapped, by Sonny Kleinfield. Atlantic–Little Brown, Boston, MA 1979.

Like It Is. Facts and Feelings About Handicaps from Kids Who Know, by Barbara Adams. Walker and Company, New York, NY, 1979.

Mealtime for People With Handicaps: A Guide for Parents and Paraprofessionals, by Nancy T. Pensis and Mary Ann Maloney. C.C. Thomas, 1983.

The Sensuous Wheeler, Multi-media Resource Center, 540 Powell Street, San Francisco, CA 94108.

Toward Intimacy and Within Reach. Human Resources Press, 72 Fifth Avenue, New York, NY 10011.

The Wheelchair in the Kitchen. Paralyzed Veterans of America, 7325 Wisconsin Avenue, Washington, DC 20014. Offers tips for designing and modifying kitchens along with safety ideas and appliance suggestions.

Wheelchair Gourmet, by Mary E. Blakeslee. Beaufort Banks, NY, 1981. A cookbook for the disabled.

CHAPTER VIII

Travel for Business and Pleasure

PUBLIC TRANSPORTATION

Getting Around in Town

The intent of the law was clearly to make all forms of public transportation completely accessible to everyone including those in wheelchairs. Although, for various reasons explained in Chapter VII, the transbus is behind schedule, a number of cities and towns have been working on the problem. For example, the metropolitan Washington D.C. area began a limited program of operating "kneeling buses" on July 1, 1979. Santa Clara County in California also has a limited program, and there are many others.

The Department of Transportation states that when a transit operator cannot provide accessibility within three years, it must provide interim service that is comparable to mainline transit service. The type of service should be developed in consultation with the handicapped community and may utilize buses, vans, taxis, or smaller buses.

One excellent way to find out about travel in your area is to keep in touch with one or another of the organizations that are working for improved transportation for the handicapped. They often put out newsletters. Special bus services are usually announced in local newspapers, although it is easy to miss what is often a one-time announcement. For the latest information check with at least one of the following: your local transportation agency, your rehabilitation counseling agency, the Easter Seal Society, the Paralyzed Veterans Association, or a health agency concerned with your particular handicap. A list of regional offices for these can be found in the Appendix.

Handicapped people have waited too long for adequate public transportation. Your frustration is fully understandable. Yet before there were any special facilities on the planning boards, some handicapped people managed to get where they were going by public transportation.

Dawnell Cruze, a blind social worker who works in Portsmouth, Virginia, admits, "I've been riding city buses since my junior year in high school." That was the year she had a summer job with the Post Office. Today, Dawnell works for the Tidewater Chapter of the American Red Cross. The trip from her home in Cradock, Virginia, to Norfolk (across the river from Portsmouth) takes about an hour. This includes one transfer to the Elizabeth River Tunnel to Norfolk, where her supervisor picks her up and drives her to work. She catches the first bus every morning at about 7:10 A.M.

Paul Filipus worked as a civil engineer in the construction industry until he was blinded in an automobile accident. Since then he has been rehabilitated and learned a new line of work. He is a computer programmer for Miles Laboratories in Elkhart, Indiana. In a report to *Chemical Technology,* a professional journal, he has this to say about transportation problems: "I have found most public transportation workers helpful and have had little trouble using taxicabs, buses, and planes. Most blind people should be able to get to and from their place of employment with a minimum of difficulty."

Selma Sack, who is now in a wheelchair because of multiple sclerosis, explored one of the transportation options available to her in the San Diego area. Her trip was for both pleasure and enlightenment. For Selma, it was also a real adventure. She lives in El Cajon, California, and depends mostly on taxicabs. One day, while talking to a cabbie, she said, "Too bad this Yellow Cab doesn't go all the way down to San Diego, since there are so many interesting things I would like to see there."

"If you really want to go alone," said the driver, "it can be done, but you have to make a special effort." The next day Selma called the Bus Transportation Corporation of San Diego and made an appointment to meet bus number 7, which has a wheelchair lift. She left home at 11:45 A.M. and took her usual Yellow Cab to the pick-up point for the Dial-A-Ride cab, which would take her to the special bus. The Dial-A-Ride cabbie told her that the fare was 65 cents one way but that that included a transfer pass to use on the special bus to San Diego.

Her trip had gone so smoothly up to that point that she had a forty-minute wait for the 1:00 P.M. bus. In a recent *Rehabilitation Gazette,* Selma described the process of boarding the bus using the wheelchair lift. When she presented her pass and was assured there was no additional fee, she was almost overwhelmed. "I am glad that I wore my dark sunglasses as it hid the tears. This is the first time in ten years that I have been able to ride in a public bus." A friendly pedestrian offered to push her the two short blocks from the bus stop to the Zoo. She arrived home later the same afternoon with the sure knowledge that she would be able to go more places in the months to come.

Intercity Transportation

The status of travel for the handicapped who need to travel for longer distances is about the same as it is for in-city transportation. The Department of Transportation now says that at least one Amtrak railroad station in each major metropolitan area and any station outside metropolitan areas and not within 50 miles of another accessible station must be made accessible. The remaining stations will be made accessible within ten years.

Within five years there will be on each passenger train at least one coach car and at least one food service car that is accessible, or the handicapped will be provided food service in their seats.

Eventually all stations have to provide telephones with sound control and telewriter equipment for those with hearing impairments. All new Amtrak stations will be completely accessible.

Travel by Air

Itzhak Perlman, the world-renowned violinist, was stricken by polio in childhood. In a recent article he relates the discomforts faced by handicapped travelers. In addition to being a great violinist, Perlman is one of the world's most experienced wheelchair travelers. "In my work it is necessary to travel almost constantly and to make countless precisely timed arrivals and departures. Like most disabled people, I am always more or less anxious about how I am going to get where I am going during the allotted travel time," he said, then added, "The entire transportation chain—cars, taxis, trains, buses, and airplanes— is designed as though everyone in the world were young and fleet of foot."

As most handicapped persons have discovered, the airlines have special regulations for handicapped persons who want to fly. There are no federal regulations specifically governing the transportation of handicapped people, by air or any other means. Individual airlines have established their own regulations in conformity with a provision of the Federal Aviation Act of 1958. This law permits the airlines to deny passage to anyone whose presence might be "inimical" to flight safety.

An issue currently in contention between blind people and the airlines is whether they should be allowed to take aboard with them the long white canes so essential to their moving about. The airlines forbid them on grounds that they would be a safety hazard by becoming projectiles in the cabin during periods of air turbulence or during an accident.

Although the airlines meet regularly to work out a uniform set of regulations governing the handicapped, they have not yet come to an agreement. This means that if you are taking a trip involving more than one airline, you need to check out the regulations on all of them to avoid being hung up somewhere along the way. In general, you may encounter three types of restrictions. None or all three of these may be applied, depending upon the individual airline's policy.

1. A medical certificate attesting to the person's health and ability to travel may be required.

2. A quota may be set on the number of wheelchairs allowed on any particular flight. This is based on the size of the aircraft, number of exits, and number of flight attendants.

3. A companion or attendant may be required to accompany a handicapped passenger.

As with all other areas regarding the rights of handicapped people, barriers are being removed. Regulations are being changed so frequently that the only sure way to know about a given flight is to check with the airline. Also check any needed airport facilities along your route. A publication that can help you to do this is listed in the resources section.

Some of the recent and not so recent changes that make air travel possible for more handicapped people are the following:

- In 1938 United Airlines was the first to rule that a Seeing Eye dog may accompany his or her master or mistress aboard a plane.
- More recently, United and Western Airlines both permitted hearing dog guides in passenger compartments.
- Frontier Airlines provides emergency procedure instructions in braille.
- TWA is the first airline to provide a wheelchair lift at airports that do not have jetways.

In these days when some changes seem to come too slowly, it is good to remember that some handicapped travelers, like Itzhak Perlman and Lina Padilla managed to travel extensively before any such changes. Lina, whom you met in Chapter V, went half way around the world with her two Peace Corps friends. It was the first vacation she ever had away from her family. It never would have been possible without her friends, who were willing and able to carry Lina, wheelchair and all, to the top of the Acropolis in Athens, as well as to other places along their route.

DRIVING YOUR OWN CAR

Learning to Drive

Most teenagers, including many handicapped teenagers, can't wait until they are old enough to drive a car. It is an undisputed mark of maturity. Many mothers welcome the event as a relief from their role as chauffeur. Many fathers view it apprehensively because the insurance rates go up on the addition of a teenage driver.

The importance of private transportation to the lives of Americans is impossible to overemphasize these days. Handicapped persons often rely even more heavily on private transportation because public transportation is inaccessible to them.

If you have not yet learned to drive, you will need to find a good training program. Check first with the driver education department of your school, which should make the course available to handicapped students. If your school does not have an adequate program, look into the qualifications of the driver training schools listed in the Yellow Pages under "Driving Instruction." You may save time by asking your rehabilitation counselor or your guidance counselor to recommend a school. A call to the nearest office of the State Motor Vehicle Department may also give you the needed information. You can also write to the State Department of Education, Driver Education Branch.

One book that is a virtual Bible on the subject of driving your own car although handicapped is *The Handicapped Driver's Mobility Guide,* published by the American Automobile Association.

It is also encouraging to know that there are now three rental car companies that rent cars with hand controls. (See the resources section.)

One Woman's Success Story

Nearly all handicapped people except those with blindness or epilepsy are permitted to obtain driver's licenses. If you feel uncertain about whether you want to or can learn to drive, take heart from the many thousands of handicapped people who drive automobiles with hand controls. There is no typical handicapped driver, of course. In fact, there is no such thing as a "typical" driver. Each person has a different story to tell about how he or she learned to drive. But we would like to tell you the story of one handicapped driver. You have met *Birdie Minor* several times before in this book. She is the speech pathologist in Fishersville, Virginia. Here, in her own words, is her story:

"I didn't begin to drive until after I had finished college and was into my career. Prior to that time, I had no idea that I would be able to drive because of my upper extremity involvement. Then I saw a quadraplegic drive and began to ask myself 'Why can't I?' I got no encouragement whatsoever. In fact, I got discouragement from fellow workers and the driving instructor where I worked.

"My brother, Ed, and his friend Mr. Ferguson, a hand control dealer in Richmond, Virginia, were the only ones who supported me. Hand controls were installed in my brother's car, and I practiced on weekends. When I realized I could drive, I bought a T-Bird and had the hand controls transferred from Ed's car. Mr. Ferguson had made a deal with me that if I could drive my brother's car, he would transfer them without charge, and he did.

"I practiced for and obtained a license in my own car. Parallel parking was one tough requirement for passing the test. I took forever to learn parallel parking. I practiced endlessly at the Division of Motor Vehicles where I would take the road test. I couldn't see the stakes between which I was supposed to park, so I used a nearby fence post and lined it up with the center of my hood. One day I finally decided I had learned to parallel park well enough to pass the test. I was in for a surprise. They had moved the stakes, but miraculously, I passed. That day was just a few days before I was to renew my learner's permit for the fourth time. A permit was for 90 days and could be renewed indefinitely. I had used nearly 270 days.

"Today, I drive a van with a wheelchair lift, from my wheelchair. The van also has a toilet and a bed for when I go camping or take long trips. These can be modified into passenger seats for everyday use. I really enjoy it!"

TRAVEL AGENCIES AND GUIDEBOOKS

Travel Agencies for the Handicapped

Traveling for recreation or business is still not easy for handicapped people, including teenagers. However, there now are many more travel agencies that specialize in planning vacations and tours for the handicapped. You will find a list of them in the resources section at the end of this chapter.

Regular Tourist Agencies

Every year the Ringling Brothers, Barnum and Bailey Circus puts on a special performance for handicapped people in the Washington D.C. area. Each of the organizations serving the handicapped is permitted to send a certain number of children along with the parents or attendants they need. Were it not for this generous gesture, most of these children and many of their parents would never see the circus. Yet some of the older children admit that there is something depressing about this huge assembly of handicapped people.

Many disabled people prefer not to go on a tour or vacation planned exclusively for groups of handicapped persons. "That puts us back in our own special world," they say. In effect, it is just the reverse of "mainstreaming." In the general population there is only a handicapped person every here and there. Many handicapped persons seek to be a part of this broader picture, rather than a member of a special group.

If this is the way you feel, you are free to work through an ordinary tourist agency. Most do an excellent job of finding ways to provide for the special needs of their customers. A woman was temporarily disabled in the early stages of a tour through Europe. Her travel agent helped her locate rental wheelchairs and accessibility guides to the cities on the tour. They even helped her check out the accessibility of the museums and art galleries she wished to visit. Whether or not you work through one of the agencies that specialize in travel plans for the handicapped, one thing is sure. Your needs will not be met unless you are absolutely candid with the travel agent. He or she must understand in what ways your needs are different from the nonhandicapped traveler.

Accessibility Guidebooks

An ever increasing number of cities and tourist attractions are publishing accessibility guides. However, it is often difficult to locate the one you need, and occasionally the guides are incomplete or out of date. This may be because they are published by such a wide variety of sponsors. Some are sponsored by private agencies. The various chapters of the Easter Seal Society have published many. Other health and rehabilitation agencies have published them. Some cities have published their own, but many seem intended chiefly to help the city's own handicapped people to move around more freely.

Because of the wide variety of sponsorship, there is little uniformity in what the guidebooks contain or in how they are organized. For example, one from a South Carolina city lists on the first page the

Alcoholic Beverage Control sales outlet stores; this turns out to be because ABC comes first alphabetically. A guide for New Orleans lists "Night Spots." Probably guides from cities that permit gambling list the major gambling establishments. A new, quite comprehensive guide to Washington D.C. lists almost all tourist attractions, monuments, and so on under "Public Buildings." Nearly all the guidebooks include something about transportation, public buildings, and other tourist attractions. Most also cover to some degree motels, hotels, restaurants, theaters, and sports arenas. Some cover office buildings. Their degree of thoroughness also varies. You may find, for example, that one book covers the accessibility of a hotel lobby and the number of rooms that are accessible to persons in wheelchairs, but it may give incomplete coverage of the public rest-room facilities on the lobby or convention floors. The guides vary widely as to whether they disclose the availability of braille signs or communications equipment for the deaf.

A guidebook that is perfectly adequate for a person with one kind of handicap may be of little use to a person with another kind of handicap. The books must be read with their limitations in mind.

Since there are literally thousands of these special guides for handicapped persons, we are unable to include even a token list in this book. You will find a number of suggestions on finding the guide books you are interested in in the resources section.

SOME DIFFERENT VACATION SUGGESTIONS

Resorts

Tourist agencies also plan other types of vacations for you, such as ones at special resorts in the mountains or at the beach. One such agency, Pinetree Tours, arranges for special buses that transport a number of wheelchair people to vacation sites. The Centers for the Handicapped, in the Washington D.C. area, plans many special vacations for handicapped adults and children.

Jim Brunotte, whom you met in the Introduction, operates a recreational ranch for handicapped persons. Although this is the only such special facility that has come to our attention, no doubt others are under development. For addresses of agencies and sources of other vacation ideas, see the resources section. Some of the resources for Chapter IX on sports may also help.

Camping

Camping is an increasingly popular vacation choice for American families. It is relatively inexpensive. Many campgrounds are available

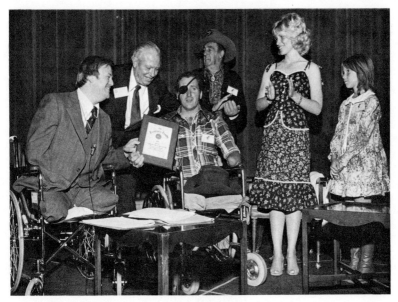

Jim Brunotte

in state and national parks and forests. The National Park Service provides information on these.

The Boy Scout and Girl Scout organizations now include handicapped young people in their camping programs. The Easter Seal Societies operate many camps for handicapped children throughout the country. All of these organizations would be good sources of information on camping opportunities for adults and families.

Amusement Parks

Many of the newest amusement parks have been built with the needs of the handicapped in mind. These include among others Busch Gardens at Williamsburg, Virginia; Kings Dominion near Richmond, Virginia, and Disney World in Florida. Although not all the rides are suitable for all handicapped persons, in general the parks are accessible.

National Parks and Monuments

A comprehensive "Guide to the National Parks and Monuments for Handicapped Tourists" is available from the President's Committee. There is also a guide to "Highway Rest Area Facilities." These publications state frankly what is and is not accessible, and to what degree. The travel guides to special cities for the handicapped usually give the needed information about tourist attractions in their areas. More information and addresses for the above are listed in the resources section.

CONCLUSION

"Paralyzed for Life, He Explores Living," reads the headline of a story in the local paper about *Gene Williams,* whom you read about at the end of the last chapter. A continuation of the story on an inside page reads "Man Seeks How and Why to Live." Now, as you are in the midst of planning your career and your life-style, is the time to "explore living" and make at least tentative decisions on "how and why to live." As you do you will discover the many and diverse ways that travel and transportation can fit into your future.

SELECTED RESOURCES CHAPTER VIII—TRANS- PORTATION

Notes: Information has been listed in the order the subjects were discussed earlier in this chapter.

Some listed publications are free, some cost a little, and some are expensive. Ask the price or include a line saying "Send only if it costs less than $1.00 or $5.00" or whatever.

* indicates books that can usually be found in public libraries or in your guidance or rehabilitation counselor's office.

PUBLIC TRANSPORTATION

Access Travel: A Guide to Accessibility of Airport Terminals. Lists design features, facilities, and services in airports across the country. Access America, Washington, DC 20202.

Access Amtrak: A Guide to Amtrak Services for Elderly and Handicapped Travelers. Office of Customer Relations, Amtrak, P.O. Box 2709, Washington, DC 20013, or call the toll-free number (800) USA-RAIL.

Buses: Greyhound Lines, Section S, Greyhound Tower, Phoenix, AZ 85077, and Continental Trailways, 1512 Commerce, Suite 500, Dallas, TX 75201.

DRIVING

Hand Controls and Assistive Devices for the Physically Disabled Driver, by J. Dillon, E.C. Colverd, and M. Less. The National Center on Employment of the Handicapped at Human Resources Center, I.U. Willets Road, Albertson, NY 11507.

The Handicapped Driver's Mobility Guide. Available at local AAA offices or write Traffic Safety Department, American Automobile Association, 8111 Gatehouse Road, Falls Church, VA 22407.

Highway Rest Areas for Handicapped Travelers. President's Committee on Employment of the Handicapped, Washington, DC 20210. Lists over 800 rest areas across the country.

Rental Cars. Avis (800) 331-1212, Hertz (800) 654-3131.

TRAVEL AGENCIES AND TOUR ORGANIZERS

Evergreen Travel, 19505L 44th Avenue West, Lynwood, WA 98036; (206) 776-1184.

Flying Wheels Tours, 143 West Bridge Street, P.O. Box 382, Owatonna, MN 55060; (507) 451-5005, or toll-free (800) 533-0363.

The Guided Tour, 555 Ashborn Road, Elkins Park, PA 19117; (215) 782-1370.

Handy-Cap Horizons, 3250 East Loretta Drive, Indianapolis, IN 46222; (317) 784-5777.

Happy Holiday Travel, 2550 N.E. 15th Avenue, Wilton Manors, Fort Lauderdale, FL 33305; (305) 561-5602.

Incentive Tours America, 12077 Wilshire Boulevard, Suite 556, West Los Angeles, CA 90025; (213) 826-2661.

Rambling Tours, Inc., P.O. Box 1304, Hallandale, FL 33009; (305) 456-2161.

Whole Person Tours, Inc., 137 West 32nd Street, Bayonne, NJ 07002; (201) 858-3400.

TRAVEL GUIDEBOOKS FOR THE HANDICAPPED

List of Guidebooks for Handicapped Travelers. Free from the President's Committee on Employment of the Handicapped, 1111 20th Street, NW, Washington, DC 20210.

International Directory of Access Guides. An aid for disabled and elderly travelers. Rehabilitation International USA, Travel Survey Department, 1123 Broadway, Room 704, New York, NY 10010, free.

To find guidebooks for any geographical area in which you are interested, check the following:

1. The nearest Information for the Handicapped Office (for a list of regional offices, see the Appendix).
2. The nearest Easter Seal Society Office locate the local office through the phone book.
3. The nearest office of the society that serves persons with your handicap.
4. The tourist council for your own city may know how to contact similar groups in other parts of the country.
5. The chambers of commerce often have an office concerned with attracting tourists. The chamber for your town may help you locate such groups in other cities.

TRAVEL BOOKS AND PUBLICATIONS

Access to the World—Travel Guide for the Handicapped. Chatham Square Press. New York, NY, 1977.

Frommer's Guide for the Disabled Traveler, the United States, Canada and Europe, by Frances Barish, 1984. Frommer/Pasmantier Publishers, Division of Simon and Schuster, Inc., 1230 Avenue of the Americas, New York, NY 10020. A comprehensive and clear guide on accessibility, tours, and everything one needs to know in the states and in Europe. $10.95.

The Itinerary, P.O. Box 1084, Bayonne, NJ 07002-1084. A monthly magazine that portrays other people's travels.

Travel-Ability—A Guide for Physically Disabled Travelers in the United States, 1978 rev. ed. Gives complete travel advice on every aspect of vacationing. Macmillan Publishing Co., New York, NY 10002.

Travel Guide for the Disabled: Western Europe, by Mary Meister Walzer, 1982. Van Nostrand Reinhold Co., 135 West 50th Street, New York, NY 10020.

FOR TRAVEL INFORMATION

Accent on Information, P.O. Box 700, Bloomington, IL 61701;

(309) 378-2961. Has a computerized retrieval system containing information on traveling and touring.

Rehabilitation International USA, 25 East 21st St., New York, NY 10010; (212) 620-4040. Has a primary purpose of serving handicapped foreign visitors, but information is also available to handicapped Americans.

Society for the Advancement of Travel for the Handicapped, 26 Court Street, Brooklyn, NY 11242; (212) 858–5483. Houses information dealing with travel services and facilities available to handicapped travelers.

Travel Information Center, Moss Rehabilitation Hospital, 12th Street and Tabor Road, Philadelphia, PA 19141; (215) 329-5715. Provides information on accessibility of hotels, airports, and other places of interest.

CHAPTER IX

A Time for Play—The Fusion of Work and Leisure

"To every thing there is a season, and a time to every purpose under the heaven." There is a time for work and a time for "play." A time for . . . The Bible does not pair the words "work" and "play" in the long series of there-is-a-time-fors that follow this verse in the Book of Ecclesiastes, but the idea comes through. "All work and no play makes Jack a dull boy," goes a time-worn saying. What it really is saying is, "Don't become a workaholic." There is much more to a creative life than working all the time.

More and more of today's young people, including disabled young people, are choosing careers from among the aptitude areas that give them the greatest satisfaction and pleasure. Many who are well matched to their life work scarcely know the difference between working and playing. The disabled young people who are most in tune with the times are achieving a fusion between their work and leisure lives that makes life more meaningful. Still, there should be a time for doing something entirely different. Even the most enthusiastic worker recognizes that "to get away from it all" is essential once in a while.

Over the millennia, mankind has developed thousands of ways to play. One person's "play" is often another person's "work," as is the case of professional athletes, artists, and performers of all kinds. The line has never been clearly drawn. In this chapter we shall discuss two broad families of recreational activities—sports and the arts. For most Americans, being a spectator of, or a participant in, one or more of the sports and one or more of the arts is a way of life. This is no less true for disabled teenagers.

SPORTS FOR FUN AND FITNESS

Both active and spectator sports are very much a part of most Americans' life-styles. The choices you have as a handicapped person are much wider than you may think. Here are some examples:

Terry Cutright of Harrisonburg, Virginia, was fifteen when doctors discovered she had curvature of the spine. Although wearing a chin-to-thigh "Milwaukee brace," she continued to be a member of her high school's track team. She was far from last in every event she entered. She did especially well in the 220-yard and the 100-yard events.

Not long after an accident put all-around athlete *Lisa Gardner* of Virginia into a wheelchair at the age of thirteen, she was once again winning medals for her swimming in the National Wheelchair Games.

Blinded by a mid-life accident, *Fred Sigert* enjoys skiing with a sighted companion at Vail, Colorado.

Avid sportswoman *Lori Merrill* of Idaho Falls, Idaho, swims, drives a snowmobile, and enjoys floating down the Snake River on a rubber raft. Lori has a rare spinal disease that has put her into a wheelchair.

Greg Simms of Culpepper, Virginia, who was severely injured in a high school football accident when he was fourteen, learned to lift 30-pound weights with each leg as he gradually regained his ability to walk.

Birdie Minor of Fishersville, Virginia, won the National Ping Pong Championship at the 17th National Wheelchair Games. She also received the Jack Gearhard Award given by the Paralyzed Veterans of America. She was the first woman ever to receive this award.

Dennis Joyner, a triple amputee from the Vietnam War, competed in the javelin throw, Ping Pong, and shot put in the Pennsylvania Wheelchair Olympics.

The Paralyzed Veterans of America published an excellent brochure on "Competitive and Recreational Wheelchair Sports." It covers archery, all-terrain vehicles, camping, swimming, boating, football, running, scuba diving, basketball, tennis, table tennis, weight lifting, and golf. You can probably find a disabled person somewhere in the world engaging in every known sport. This is true, however, only if you consider "the handicapped" as a class. But you can't do that, because every person is unique. The selection of and pursuit of a sport by any person depends on many things—height, weight, sight, hearing, mobility, strength, coordination, and, most important of all, personal preference.

Growing Interest in Sports

Fifty years ago the average American gave little time or thought to participating in active sports. Those who had jobs during the great depression usually had more than enough chores to do at home to

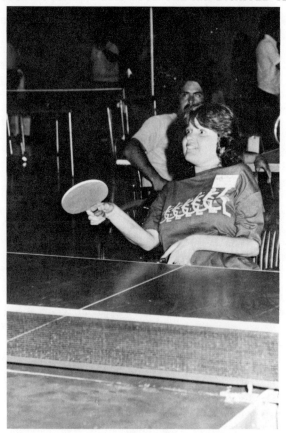

Birdie Minor

fill their spare time and use up their remaining energy. The unemployed often put in long hours of hard work in more menial jobs than they had ever done. The average homemaker was quick to point out that the amount of physical energy she used and the exercise she got was more than enough! "Who has time for sports?" she might say contemptuously. "They are for the members of country clubs and the very rich who have more time and money than they know what to do with!"

But times have changed. We are in the midst of a great surge of participant interest in active sports. This interest is mainly the result of research findings that the body functions better and lives longer if it is regularly exercised. The best kind of exercise, the researchers tell us, is one that exercises the heart and breathing muscles. Disabled teenagers' bodies have the same need for exercise, although different ways of achieving it may have to be worked out.

Competitive sports for the disabled in the United States were initiated over thirty years ago with wheelchair basketball and bowling. By now several organizations are deeply involved in sponsoring competitive sporting events. They establish the classifications fairly so that people with many kinds of handicaps can compete in many sports. See the resources section at the end of this chapter for sources of information.

ABOUT THE FUN PART

We have just explained the sports for fitness part—that is, the need to exercise your cardiovascular system. What about the fun part? If you are not athletically inclined, you may never have experienced the joy of physical activity. Your reaction to competition may be to avoid it completely. This is understandable after years of being ruled out of the competitions by rules made for and by "normal" people. But if you can compete against others who are more nearly your physical equals, you may find your appetite for competition sharpened. You may find that you love it.

It was a last-minute idea when *Birdie Minor* signed up for the Ping Pong competition in the National Wheelchair Games. Like most disabled people, she had had little experience at winning anything even slightly athletic. But she *won* the Ping Pong tournament. She was "excited and delighted." "It was unbelievable," she said. "I really surprised myself by winning. Most paraplegics would probably do better in the games than they think they would if they would only enter. I had no idea that I could win until I played someone in my own class."

Thomas Lyczko is the profoundly deaf college student you read about in Chapter IV. In explaining what sports mean to him he said, "One of the most important activities in my life is distance running. I run three to ten miles daily. Since I started running in 1974, I have become convinced that despite the aches and pains involved, it is one of the best things there is. It makes me feel good mentally and physically. I enjoy it. I think it has helped me with my schoolwork. I believe running has improved my confidence a little, and that helps me keep my head together. Running has afforded me a number of unique experiences and achievements. It has helped me to meet many people and make some good friends. One of the highlights of 1978 was training ten miles a day during October. This was in preparation for the New York City Marathon. It is really indescribable how you feel during the marathon—being carried along by the enthusiasm of the crowd. All in all, running is a lot of fun and worth the trouble it takes."

Try as many different kinds of sports as you can arrange. You may find yourself becoming excited about a whole new area of activities that you never thought about. You may find a new delight in competition. You may find a new joy in fellowship with other sportsmen and sportswomen, and a new avenue toward making friends.

Spectator Sports

For every person who is active in sports, there are hundreds who are active spectators. They learn all about the sport, attend the games, and cheer for the participants. They join fan clubs. They discuss events and techniques with other spectator sportsmen. Sports become both a focal interest and a means of socializing with friends. It can well be said that spectators are as important to sports as are the players. The "big" sports are not those with the greatest number of participants, but the ones with the largest number of spectators. In sports there is a role for everyone, professional participant and spectator alike. Go out and enjoy.

THE ARTS AND YOUR LIFE-STYLE

In addition to engaging in sports for fun and fitness, many Americans choose to spend a part of their free time on a hobby or other recreational activity chosen from the fine arts or the folk arts. "The arts" is a high-sounding term, and it is not broad enough to cover all the activities included in this discussion. As we see it, "the arts" include everything from oil painting to quilting and from wood carving to playing in a string quartet.

Connoisseurs, Collectors, and Hobbyists

As in sports, you can be a "spectator artist" as well as a practitioner of the art. Some persons become experts on art. They spend a lot of time in art galleries. They read books, attend lectures, go to colleges and universities and take courses in the area of their interest. We call them connoisseurs. No matter how expert they become, they are still spectator artists.

Connoisseurs frequently become collectors. Paul Mellon and family members before him were connoisseurs of art with enough money to buy many valuable paintings. These are now the basis of the National Gallery of Art in Washington, D.C. Most collections are not so vast or so expensive. People can and do enjoy collecting almost anything— posters, baseball cards, beer cans, buttons, depression glass, antique furniture, stamps, coins, campaign buttons, records by one or many artists, and on and on. One might rightly say my hobby is collecting this or that. The dictionary defines a hobby as an activity engaged in purely for pleasure.

A very large percentage of hobbies involve making something. Here again the range is endless—from cabinetmaking, embroidery, or macramé to flower arranging, gardening, piano playing, or oil painting. The person who takes up oil painting may learn a lot about it but not become a connoisseur. The thrust of his or her interest is in actually painting in oils on canvas. There are no rules against becoming all three at the same time. Many persons become connoisseurs, collectors, and hobbyists all centered around the same interest area.

What turns you on, gives you the purest pleasure? You may already be started on one or more hobbies. If not, now is the time to try out some new areas.

The Arts and Your Communications Skills

The arts provide a variety of ways for us to communicate with our fellow human beings, ways that do not depend on words and language. This is of particular interest to persons who are language-disabled. Some of the ways this gap can be filled through art are seen in the following stories.

Ann Riordan teaches dance at the University of Utah. She is also trained in special education. She works with groups of handicapped people who wish to explore the world of dance and movement. One group she taught at the Work Activities Center for Handicapped Adults in Salt Lake City included thirty or so handicapped persons, some twelve of them in wheelchairs. Their ages ranged from twenty-one to fifty. The range of handicap on a trainable level included Down's syndrome, cerebral palsy, other forms of brain damage and retardation, and various levels of emotional problems.

Mrs. Riordan, who worked with this group for more than two years, says, "Their enthusiasm for movement was overwhelming. They excited me as I excited them. We found a mutual exchange and sharing through the movement experience. From this basic group there developed a performing group of twelve students. These students have the stage presence, creative personality, repertory, and aesthetic qualities found in many modern dance companies." In evaluating the experience she says, "These people seem to have changed. They seem proud of their group, feel beautiful, and have something unique to give to someone else. They can create dances and relate through movement to each other. They can control their own bodies—they can dance!"

Andrew Stamm, whom you read about in Chapter IV, is a severely retarded young man who enjoys taking part in both sports and the arts. In 1974, 1975, and 1976 he ran and won the one-mile race in the Washington State Special Olympics. He also swims, hikes, and goes on long bike trips. His art work has been featured at Washington State's Very Special Arts Fair. He has demonstrated his sculpturing techniques at the Arts for the Handicapped show. These are only his more recent art achievements. There are over 100 paintings by Andrew framed and hanging.

Susan Arch is the Coordinator of the Expressive Arts Program at Western Pennsylvania School for the Blind. This is a program to provide children with experiences in art, drama, and movement. The aim is to develop the children's creativity and capacity for self-expression. After more than five years' experience with the program, Susan concludes that, "The children have creative spirits that can find fulfillment in art. They show great pleasure in the use of materials and have ideas they wish to give form to. . . . Finally, the involvement in art can enhance the children's growth in other areas. Because having a good feeling about reaching out and being curious about materials and objects is extremely important for the partially sighted and the totally blind child in learning to read braille and in acquiring mobility and self-care skills."

Art for Fun and Profit

For many people who have developed their talents, practicing their art becomes a career. For *Fred Mancuso,* Canadian landscape artist whom you read about in Chapter II, painting began as an avocation and finally became a full-time career.

Another painter who classifies himself as a "painter by foot" is *Edward Kwiatkowski* of Holyoke, Massachusetts. He was born with cerebral palsy affecting his upper limbs, so he uses his right foot. It takes him about three weeks to complete a painting. His work has appeared in more than twenty exhibits in as many years.

Joni Eareckson (Chapter I) paints and writes her books using a mouth stick. Like many others who have been severely injured, she found the beginnings of her new career in the long hours spent in rehabilitation.

Ed Walker, blind disc jockey and talk-show host (Chapter II), has become something of an expert on popular music of the 1920's, 1930's, and 1940's. This serves him well in his career. He also enjoys attending live performances and has built an extensive record collection.

These are but a very few examples of handicapped persons who have discovered and developed talents that could later be used in profit-making activities. People who are working in areas that give them the most satisfaction and pleasure are among the happiest and the luckiest in the world.

National Committee *Arts for the Handicapped

Special programs for art for the handicapped have just begun to be developed. They are not as prevalent or as available as services offered by the rehabilitation agencies, which were started many years ago. The National Committee *Arts for the Handicapped is the first national effort along these lines. It began only in 1974.

The Committee's principal interest is in stimulating more and better art education for handicapped school-age children. According to Wendy Parks, Executive Director, the major effort has been to communicate "a single message to many thousands of teachers, parents, administrators, and artists in each of the fifty states. The arts are powerful vehicles for enhancing learning and enriching living for all handicapped children." The Committee finds that only a small percentage of the estimated millions of handicapped children in the U.S. receive any art education. If children never have an opportunity to learn about the arts or to experience them, they will have little interest in them as adults.

The National Committee sponsors some pilot projects in art education. They have stimulated many of the Very Special Arts Fairs being held across the country. They have a vast network of contacts in the arts and are an excellent source of pertinent information.

Another good source is the *National Arts and the Handicapped Information Service*. This is made possible through a grant from the National Endowment for the Arts—a federal agency—and the Educational Facilities Laboratory of New York. You will find the addresses for both these organizations listed in the resources section at the end of this chapter.

COMMUNITY RECREATION PROGRAMS

More and more local community recreation departments are developing programs for the handicapped. At the present time, these are rather limited. Alexandria, Virginia, for example, offers a Special Olympics Sports Night program once a week for mildly handicapped teens and adults. In it, participants have an opportunity to learn skills in basketball, volleyball, floor hockey, and gymnastics. There is also a Special Olympics competition. To find out what may be offered in your community, call the recreation department.

CONCLUSION

A word needs to be said about accessibility. In order to engage in sports and enjoy concerts, museums, or theaters, one must be able to get into and use buildings. From the time of the Greeks and even before, a long flight of steps to the main entrance of a building was the architect's device to make the building more impressive. The U.S. Capitol, built in the mid-1800's, is a case in point. Unfortunately many of our public buildings have followed a similar style. These include museums, universities, libraries, art galleries, and many other tourist attractions.

The status of compliance with the new accessibility legislation was discussed in more detail in the preceding chapter. Suffice it to say that compliance to date is uneven. Much checking out of facilities will probably be necessary for a long time to come. Access depends, as it always has, on a handicapped person's determination and firm belief that, "If there's a will, there's a way."

SELECTED RESOURCES CHAPTER IX—RECREATION

Note: Information has been listed in the order the subjects were discussed earlier in this chapter.

Some listed publications are free, some cost a little, and some are expensive. Ask the price or include a line saying "Send only if it costs less than $1.00 or $5.00" or whatever.

SPORTS FOR FUN AND FITNESS

For information on specific sports:

All Terrain Vehicles: Wheelchair Motorcycle Association, 101 Torrey Street, Brockton, MA 02401.

Archery: The National Archery Association, Ronks, PA 17572, or National Wheelchair Athletic Association, 40-24 62nd Street, Woodside, NY 11377.

Basketball: National Wheelchair Basketball Association, 110 Seaton Building, University of Kentucky, Lexington, KY 40506

Boating: Handicapped Boaters Association, P.O. Box 1134, Ansonia Station, NY 10023.

Bowling: American Wheelchair Bowling Association, N54 W15858 Larkspur Lane, Menomonee Falls, WI 53051.

Cross-country skiing: Ski for Light, 1455 West Lake Street, Minneapolis, MN 55408.

Horseback riding: National Foundation For Happy Horsemanship for the Handicapped, P.O. Box 462, Malvern PA 19355.

Softball: National Wheelchair Softball Association, P.O. Box 737, Sioux Falls, SD 57101.

Table tennis, weight lifting, swimming: National Wheelchair Athletic Commission, 2107 Templeton Gap Road, Suite C, Colorado Springs, CO 80907.

Tennis: National Foundation of Wheelchair Tennis, 3857 Birch Street, Newport, CA 92660.

For additional information on sports, sports programs, and recreation (addresses given above will not be repeated):

National Easter Seal Society for Crippled Children and Adults, 2023 West Ogden Avenue, Chicago, IL 60612.

Association for Retarded Citizens, 2501 Avenue J, P.O. Box 6109, Arlington, TX 76011.

National Association of the Physically Handicapped, 76 Elm Street, London, OH 43140.

Girl Scouts of the USA, Program Management, 830 Third Avenue, New York, NY 10022.

Boy Scouts of America, Education/Handicapped Relationship Service, 1325 Walnut Hill Lane, Irving, TX 75062.

Indoor Sports Club, 1145 Highland Street, Napoleon, OH 43545.

Paralyzed Veterans of America, PVA National Building, 801 18th Street, NW, Washington, DC 20006.

Special Olympics, 1701 K Street, NW, Suite 203, Washington, DC 20006.

National Therapeutic Recreation Society, 3101 Park Center Drive, Alexandria, VA 22307.

American Alliance for Health, Physical Education, Recreation and Dance, Programs for the Handicapped, 1900 Association Drive, Reston, VA 22091.

United Cerebral Palsy Associations, Inc. (for information on competitive sports for cerebral palsied), 66 East 34th Street, New York, NY 10016, or call your local UCP chapter.

National Handicapped Sports and Recreation Association, P.O. Box 33141, Farragut Station, Washington, DC 20023.

National Association for Disabled Athletes, 80 Huguenot Avenue, Suite 11-B, Englewood, NJ 07631.

United States Association for Blind Athletes, 55 West California Avenue, Beach Haven, NJ 08008.

National Association of Sports for Cerebral Palsied, 66 East 34th Street, New York, NY 10016.

International Committee of Sports for the Deaf, Gallaudet College, Washington, DC 20002.

THE ARTS AND YOUR LIFESTYLE

National Committee, Arts for the Handicapped, Kennedy Center Education Program, J.F.K. Center for the Performing Arts, Washington, DC 20566.

National Arts and the Handicapped Information Service, Arts and Special Constituencies Project, National Endowment for the Arts, 2401 E Street, NW, Room 1200, Washington, DC 20506.

Association of Handicapped Artists, Inc., 1134 Rand Building, Buffalo, NY 14203.

Access to the Past: Museum Programs and Handicapped Visitors by Alice P. Kenney, 1980.

CHAPTER X

Reading and the Rest of Your Life

The elderly couple had given up using their dining room in favor of eating at the kitchen table. In the years since it had been used, the dining room had begun to look more like a warehouse for a paper recycling plant. Oh, it was neat enough. It was organized, too, in a way. On each chair there was a pile of magazines. Some were general circulation weeklies or monthlies. A pile of *Ladies' Home Journals* was on one, *Good Housekeeping* on another. *U.S. News, Time,* and *Newsweek* shared two chairs pushed together. A pile of *Atlantic Monthlies* were on one chair, *Consumer Reports* were on another. Three tall piles of *National Geographics* were on the floor in the corner beside the buffet. *Popular Mechanics* was piled on the other side of the buffet. On top were three or four piles of "prestige" magazines such as *Smithsonian, Americana, Early American Life,* and a journal of antiques.

The piles of newspapers on the rectangular dining room table never got too high before they were removed. There were always two or three weeks of the Sunday New York *Times,* three or four days of the local daily paper, and several weeks of the suburban weekly. Copies of the many free shoppers were generally not saved more than a week.

In the two remaining corners of the room were neat piles of professional journals that continued to come even though the couple had been retired for several years. His were engineering. Hers were elementary education. "After all," they would tell you, "we like to keep up to date in the fields where we spent so many years of our lives."

But they were not keeping up—not really. They were saving the magazines until they had time to read them, but they were months— even years—behind on some of them. They were facing the reading dilemma. It is dealt with in one way or another by all literate Americans.

131

THE READING DILEMMA

One result of the information explosion of the past fifteen years has been the proliferation of books and publications of all kinds. It is literally impossible for any one of us to read even those publications that are sent to us unrequested. Besides, there are many things we want to read for pleasure or profit. Sometimes we have to search them out in bookstores or on newsstands. Everyone makes choices. We discard some things without reading them at all. We skip much of the newspapers and certain articles in the magazines we receive. However, every conscientious person feels that he or she needs to keep current in a number of areas. Among them are the following:

Your Profession or Vocation

The increasing popularity of speed-reading courses may be directly related to the number of professors and professional and business men and women who arrive home each night with their briefcases bulging with reading they couldn't get around to in the office. The amount of reading you do that relates to your chosen career may make the difference between excelling and merely getting by. Some reading is absolutely necessary. Nevertheless, so much comes across the desks of most professional and management people that some selection is also necessary.

Try to find one or two newspapers, newsletters, or journals that cover your entire field. Select the one or two you feel do the best job. Don't waste time reading the others. Then select a limited number of publications in your own area of specialization. You may find one or two that become your favorites, and you will want to read them thoroughly. You may find others that you can browse through. Some you can merely glance at and gain a general sense of their content. If you make your selections thoughtfully and resist the temptation to try to cover everything, you will save valuable time.

The amount of reading required in the skilled trades or the arts is somewhat less, but here too, getting ahead often depends on your willingness and ability to learn through reading.

Current Events—City, State, National, and International

An informed citizenry is what makes a democracy work. Yet most of us quaver at the thought of what would be necessary to keep *really* up to date with what is going on in our town, city, and state, to say nothing of the nation and the world. The volume of what we need to know keeps growing as government bureaucracies grow and as the world becomes smaller because of improved communications.

Local newspapers usually cover local and state events in some detail.

They also give limited coverage of national and international events. Most weekly papers give more detail on small towns or suburban areas where they are published.

National newsmagazines give broad coverage to both national and international events. Certain large city newspapers like the New York *Times,* the Washington *Post,* and the Los Angeles *Times* also give in-depth coverage. Radio and television cover a broad range in their net-work news broadcasts. Because of lack of time, many important national and international events are either not covered or covered very superfi-cially.

Sample the various publications available to you. Make your selec-tions carefully. You will want to find publications that give good cover-age of the issues of personal concern to you. You will also want coverage in depth of state, national, and international issues that relate to our common future as U.S. citizens. You can broaden your viewpoint and your understanding if you are able to read a variety of publications or change those you read every few years.

The Handicapped and Your Handicap

Handicapped people are becoming better organized and more politi-cally active. You need to keep up to date in order to obtain benefits to which you may be entitled. Many suggested starting points to obtain information you need are given in the resources section for Chapter II—Career Selection and Finding Vocational Guidance, Chapter III—School Selection, Chapter IV—Financing Education, and Chapter VI—Legal Rights.

Your reading can also help you to improve your life-style. Certain starting points are given in the resources for Chapter VII on Life-style, Chapter VIII on Travel, and Chapter IX on Recreation. In addition, certain very helpful publications for the handicapped in general are listed in the resources section of this chapter.

You will also want to keep up to date on the latest medical break-throughs in the treatment or cure of your particular disability. One of the best sources for this kind of information is the voluntary associa-tion that concerns itself with helping persons with your particular handi-cap. You will find a list of the national offices of a broad range of such agencies in the Appendix. If you are unable to find a local chapter in your phone book, write to the national association. They will direct you to the nearest source of aid. Many of these associations also have special publications or newsletters concerning technological advances, legal rights, and all other problems faced by persons sharing your handi-cap.

Reading for Pleasure

We have discussed the various needs for reading that we all encounter as we go through life. Now we would like to discuss the kind of reading that is most meaningful to the individual—reading for pleasure. By now you probably know what you like to read for pleasure. You have the choice of the whole range of fiction and nonfiction.

Special-interest Reading. This is reading about a subject usually unrelated to your career, simply because you are interested. We know a young man who reads book after book about archeology the way some others read the latest mysteries or westerns. He is intrigued with the Dead Sea Scrolls and the latest digs in ancient Persia that are revealing vestiges of civilizations alluded to in the Old Testament. There are many key magazines. Ask your librarian to help you find ones in your interest area.

Others like to read about art or artists, history, science, or science fiction. Perhaps you are intrigued with man's future in space and like to read articles and books that outline how the first space colonies will work. Some people's reading relates to their hobby. Some people like poetry, novels, or books on philosophy or science. Make a list of the subjects that give you reading pleasure. It is handy to have around when people ask you what you want for Christmas.

Inspirational reading. The great religious books like the Bible and the Koran and works of philosophy and poetry fill this need for many persons. Some handicapped as well as nonhandicapped persons like to read about handicapped persons who have solved problems. There is a growing body of handicapped writers who have written their own stories. They have contributed to the pleasure and inspiration of others. There is also a great body of inspirational books, magazines, and newspapers that are often, but not always, related to one of the organized religions. Bookstores often classify this type of literature as philosophical, religious, or self-help books. It is a good department to browse in to discover your own tastes. There are also religious bookstores that usually have a broader selection of such publications.

HOW TO FIND A BOOK

In recent years we have heard and read much about "why Johnny can't read." Such articles usually cite alarming percentages of today's young people who are able to read not at all or only at the barest functional level. Despite all this, the publishing industry is alive and well and constantly growing. The demand for more and more books and publications keeps rising. There are more books about more specialized subjects than ever before.

Radio and television daytime talk shows these days are made up largely of interviews with authors of newly published books. Although the show's host usually says that the book is available at local bookstores, it is often not that easy. One of the authors of this book once accumulated a list of five or six books she had heard about on television and wished to obtain. After a phone survey of several stores and visits to the most convenient ones, she had acquired only one of the six in the several months that followed. We don't know why this is so. Book promotion schedules and the distribution channels seem not always to be well coordinated. If you hear about a book you would really like to get your hands on, we suggest this procedure.

1. Always get the complete title and the names of the author and publisher.
2. If you do not have the name of the publisher, ask your librarian to look it up in her catalog of new publications.
3. Armed with this information, call several convenient bookstores to see if they have a copy and will hold it for you. Better yet, arrange to have the store send it to you upon receipt of your check.
4. If all else fails, write to the publisher and ask whether you can order a copy direct. In order to avoid receiving a form letter directing you to the nearest bookstore, explain that you have already tried that approach.

CONCLUSION

No matter what reading preferences you develop over the years, reading for pleasure can bring much joy into your life. Some famous people discovered this many years ago. "When I am reading a book, whether wise or silly, it seems to me to be alive and talking to me," said Jonathan Swift, English satirist who died in 1745. Herbert Spencer, an English philosopher who died in 1803, had this perceptive thought: "Reading is seeing by proxy." Many agree with him—especially those who read braille rather than print.

Helen Keller was both blind and deaf from infancy. In her autobiography, *The Story of My Life,"* she wrote this about reading:

Literature is my Utopia. Here I am not disenfranchised. No barrier of the senses shuts me out from the sweet, gracious discourse of my book-friends. They talk to me without embarrassment or awkwardness.

SELECTED RESOURCES CHAPTER X—READING

Notes: Some listed publications are free, some cost a little, and some are expensive. Ask the price, or include a line saying "Send only if it costs less than $1.00 or $5.00" or whatever.

GENERAL INTEREST NEWSLETTERS AND MAGAZINES FOR THOSE WITH ALL HANDICAPS

Accent on Living, quarterly magazine. The Accent on Information, P.O. Box 700, Bloomington, IL 61701.

Disabled USA, quarterly magazine. The President's Committee on Employment of the Handicapped, 1111 20th Street, NW, #600, Washington, DC 20036.

In the Mainstream, bimonthly newsletter. Free from Mainstream, Inc., 1200 15th Street, NW, Washington, DC 20005 (also available on tape).

Rehabilitation Gazette, annual international journal. 4502 Maryland Avenue, St. Louis, MO 63108.

NAPH Newsletter, quarterly. National Association for the Physically Handicapped, 76 Elm Street, London, OH 43140.

Programs for the Handicapped, monthly. Office for Handicapped Individuals, U.S. Department of Education, Room 3631, Switzer Building, 330 C Street, SW, Washington, DC 20202.

CATALOGS AND OTHER SOURCES OF READING MATERIALS

Association of Hospital and Institutional Libraries (American Library Association pamphlet: *Reading Aids for the Handicapped*— sources for aids, large-type books and newspapers, talking books, etc.), 50 East Huron Street, Chicago, IL 60611.

Modern Talking Pictures Service, Inc. Captioned Films for the Deaf), 5000 Park Street, North, St. Petersburg, FL 33709. Lends educational and entertainment captioned films.

National Library Service for the Blind and Physically Handicapped (Magazines in Special Media). Reference Section, Library of Congress, Washington, DC 20542.

American Foundation for the Blind (catalog of publications, pamphlets on braille publishers, publishers of large-type books, etc.), 15 West 16th Street, New York, NY 10011.

American Printing House for the Blind, Instructional Materials Reference Center (hand-transcribed textbooks), 1836 Frankfort Avenue, Louisville KY 40206.

The American Council of the Blind (The Braille Forum), 190 Lattimore Road, Rochester, NY 14620.

Recording for the Blind, Inc., 20 Roszel Road, Princeton, NJ 08540. Lends taped educational textbooks at no charge.

Library of Congress, Division for the Blind and Visually Handicapped (talking books, etc.), Washington, DC 20542.

Address List: Regional and Sub-Regional Libraries for the Blind and Physically Handicapped, Library of Congress, address above.

GENERAL INTEREST MAGAZINES AND NEWSLETTERS FOR THOSE WITH SPECIAL HANDICAPS

Arthritis: *Arthritis Foundation Newsletter,* 3400 Peachtree Road, NE, Atlanta, GA 30326.

Blindness: *Talking Book Topics,* bimonthly. Division for the Blind and Physically Handicapped, Library of Congress, Washington, DC 20542.

Cerebral Palsy: *Newsletter.* United Cerebral Palsy Association, 66 East 34th Street, New York, NY 10016.

Cystic Fibrosis: *Commitment,* quarterly publication. Cystic Fibrosis Foundation, 6000 Executive Boulevard, Suite 309, Rockville, MD 20852.

Deafness: *The Deaf American,* magazine. National Association of the Deaf, 814 Thayer Street, Silver Spring, MD 20910.

Diabetes: *Newsletter.* American Diabetic Association, 600 Fifth Avenue, New York, NY 10020.

Epilepsy: *Newsletter.* Epilepsy Foundation of America, 4351 Garden City Drive, Suite 406, Landover, MD 20785.

Kidney Disease: *KF Newsletter.* National Kidney Foundation, 2 Park Avenue, New York, NY 10016.

Multiple Sclerosis: *MS Messenger,* newsletter. National Multiple Sclerosis Society, 205 East 42nd Street, New York, NY 10017.

Muscular Dystrophy: *MDA Newsletter.* Muscular Dystrophy Association of America, 810 Seventh Avenue, New York, NY 10019.

Paraplegia: *Paraplegia News,* Monthly. Paralyzed Veterans of America, 5201 North 19th Avenue, Suite 108, Phoenix AZ 85015.

Spina Bifida: *Newsletter.* 343 South Dearborn, Chicago, IL 60604.

Learning Disability: *ACLD Newsletter.* Association for Children and Adults with Learning Disabilities, 4156 Library Road, Pittsburgh, PA 15234.

BOOKS BY HANDICAPPED PEOPLE

(Note: Because of limited space, we include only books by persons who are mentioned in this book.)

David Hartman. *White Coat, White Cane.* Playboy Press, 747 Third Avenue, New York, NY, 10017, 1979.

Robert Meyers. *Like Normal People.* McGraw-Hill Book Company, New York, NY 1978.

Eareckson, Joni and Steve Estes. *A Step Further,* 2d ed. Zondervan, New York, NY.

Eareckson, Joni with Joe Musser. *Joni.* Zondervan Publishing House, Grand Rapids, MI 1976.

CHAPTER XI

Words to Live By

In this book you have met many people with many different kinds of handicaps. Undoubtedly some of them are more and some less handicapped than you are. In this chapter you will find more of the ideas and philosophies that they feel have contributed most to their success, plus a few from other handicapped persons who have not appeared earlier in this book. These words forged out of their lifetimes of living are their messages to you who are just beginning to develop patterns for successful living.

TAKE CHARGE OF YOUR LIFE

"Have as much control as possible over your own destiny, and don't live your life always to satisfy someone else."

John Kemp, Illinois lawyer
(congenital quadruple amputee)

"I try not to be governed by situations—by mere luck. I saw beyond what society says you can't do."

Gene Williams, jazz musician
(paraplegia)

"I am completely in charge of my life; even though I may have special needs, this does not deny me the right to achieve the very best I can."

Laureen Summers, Maryland designer
and weaver (cerebral palsy)

"Either you stand by the roadside and watch the world go by, or you get in there and fight."

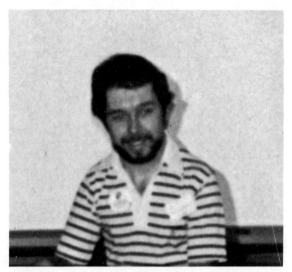

Henry Henscheid

Jim Brunotte, recreational ranch owner-operator and Handicapped American of the Year 1979 (triple amputee) quoted in *The Reader's Digest,* August, 1979

BE SELF-RELIANT

"The only real natural resource this country has is our young minds. They are to be our future lawyers, legislators, and leaders. Unfortunately, some of these young minds are put into disabled bodies. This being the case, we have to prove that we are not just equal to our peers, but in any case better than."

Captain Keith D. Heuer, co-owner and operator of a pleasure boat chartering business (double amputee)

"What everyone needs to learn mainly is personal discipline. You have to rely on yourself. You can't do without faith and discipline."

Henry Henscheid, Director of Advocacy for California Easter Seal Societies (cerebral palsy)

"No matter what happens to you, you are ultimately responsible for yourself."

Gene Williams (identified above)

BELIEVE IN YOURSELF—BE CONFIDENT

"You must believe in improving yourself first if you want others to believe in you."

Terry Hooton, Oregon, custodian
(intellectually impaired)

"Don't give up too easily. Have faith in yourself. With time and effort, things seem to fall into place."

Edward Kwiatkowski, Massachusetts
painter by foot (cerebral palsy)

BE DETERMINED—BE PERSISTENT

"Have determination and will power. Do not get discouraged easily."

Edward Kwiatkowski (identified above)

"Keep at it. Don't lose faith in your abilities. Hang in there!"

Henry Henscheid (identified above)

"I may be a limited quad, but if I set my mind to do something, I can find some way to do it!"

Steve Monroe, Virginia
computer programmer (quadraplegic)

"Don't give up—you have many rights under Sections 504 and 505."

John Kemp (identified above)

ASSESS YOUR STRENGTHS AND WEAKNESSES

"With proper support the child or adult will work on his or her strengths and learn how to work around the weaknesses. They move more quickly with the help of people who understand the problems of the learning disabled and how much can be done constructively— provided one isn't caught up in society's 'round holes in square pegs' routine."

Jo Ann Haseltine, California government worker (learning-disabled)

"Assess your strengths and weaknesses. Don't be afraid to try something new. Don't be afraid to get help."

Henry Henscheid (identified above)

STARTING AT THE BOTTOM

"Working just because the money is good is a very sad thing to do. The rule is to get into a job you enjoy, no matter how small. Being at peace with yourself as I have found is worth more than all the gold in the world."

Fred Mancuso, Canadian artist
(multiple sclerosis, diabetes,
hypertension)

"If you say you will take anything even if it's part time, chances are you will work yourself up to full time. Sometimes because of where you live or transportation problems, or your type of disability, you have no choice but to limit yourself. But if this is not the case, then don't. Handicapped people often tend to limit themselves."

Terry Hooton (identified above)

RISE TO THE CHALLENGE

"It's much better to be challenged and become strong than to have it easy and be dependent on other people for the rest of our lives."

Nick De Panfilis, Texas high
school student (vision impairment
and severe hearing impairment)

"A Bible study group has met in my home once a week for the past five years. I also read to the blind. I get around in an electric wheelchair, type with a mouth stick. Because I have been blessed with a loving family and friends, and have a strong faith in God, I can face each new day with a spirit of challenge."

Patti Burke, New York, homemaker-
artist (quadraplegia)

ALWAYS GIVE YOUR BEST

"I try to put forth the maximum effort in everything I do. I try to do everything right and fully, leaving nothing undone."

"Don't limit yourself—because others will. Insist on getting the best out of life even if you must go to a lot of trouble in getting it."

> Dave Harmon, Greenville, S.C.
> pharmacy intern (quadraplegic)

"Mainly I do try to do my best in whatever I do. I always try to enjoy myself while I'm at it, whether it's work or play."

> Thomas Lyczko, college student at
> Colgate (severely impaired hearing
> and vision)

SOME CAN-DO ATTITUDES

"I try to think more about the things I am able to do, as well as devising ways of doing things that could be a possibility for me. But as far as the things I absolutely can't do, I don't dwell on them except to reevaluate them from time to time. Times do change, and things are possible today that I wouldn't have thought possible ten years ago. Who knows what the next ten years will bring?"

> Tony Gaffney, Wisconsin, income
> tax service specialist (polio quad)

"My basic philosophy toward physical disability is that being a quadraplegic is not a tragedy, but an inconvenience perpetuated by architectural and social attitudes."

> Tedde Kast Scharf, Director of
> Services for Disabled Students
> at the University of Northern
> Colorado (muscular dystrophy)

"The question people sometimes ask me 'What can you do?' is inappropriate, for the only thing I can't do is walk."

"Never allow one's handicap to interfere with career dreams. Consider it a wonderful asset, one which cannot help but make you a bit more insightful about your life and living and getting along with others."

> Melissa Oliver, recent University
> of Virginia School of Law graduate
> (paraplegia)

"Always have a time of meditation or a quiet time for planning your day daily. This has done wonders for me. Also, always have a sense of humor."

> Birdie Minor, speech pathologist
> (polio quad)

IF PEOPLE STARE

"Don't be hurt because people look at you. You are their equal. You have worth because of your own self, and perhaps they watch you with admiration because they have never seen a person like you who goes out and lives life as they do."

> Gabriella Brimmer, writer in
> Mexico (cerebral palsy quad)

DON'T BE BITTER

Williams decided to pass up a chance for a major lawsuit against St. Albans or his wrestling coach. "A lot of people think I was stupid not to do that . . . but who was I going to sue really?" In thinking it through, he came to the conclusion that he should have had his neck X-rayed long before it was hurt, since it had been hurt some time before in a football game. "I ignored a fundamental warning signal."

> Gene Williams (identified above)

ON SUFFERING

"To be alive is to suffer sometimes. Suffering isn't all there is to life, but unless we accept misery as an integral part of it, all other experiences are diminished."

> Ann Sayers, wife of Bill Sayers,
> writer (polio respiratory quad)
> from an article in *Guideposts,*
> October, 1977.

"Today as I look back, I am convinced that the whole ordeal of my paralysis was inspired by God's love. I wasn't the brunt of some cruel divine joke. God has *reasons* behind my suffering, and learning some of them has made all the difference in the world."

> Joni Eareckson, writer (quadraplegia),
> from the dust cover of
> her new book with Steve Estes,
> *A Step Further.*

THE "WHY ME" QUESTION

There is probably no answer to this question that every handicapped person asks himself or herself sooner or later. But many handicapped persons have found their own satisfactory answers like the one below:

"I must admit that if the pointing finger of God punched through the clouds and a voice boomed 'Listen kid, I'm going to do you a big favor and strike you with polio today,' I'd be the first to exclaim ad nauseam, 'Why me?'

"As I look back now from this pinnacle of survival, I see that my husband, children, and I have maneuvered through an era of turmoil that destroyed many families. Perhaps we survived and flourished because my polio was a buffer, an object of intense concern, that served as an adhesive to hold our family together."

> Mary Ann Hamilton, owner of a
> toy store in Denver (respiratory
> polio quad)

ON MEMBERSHIP IN A VERY SPECIAL GROUP

Many persons newly handicapped by accident or illness do not readily accept their membership in what for them is a new group—the handicapped. It was fifteen years after Patricia Karn acquired multiple sclerosis before she was able to write:

"In 1970 I was invited to attend a class for multiple sclerosis patients sponsored by the San Diego Community Colleges. I joined the group and learned to be aware of a new community of the disabled. We are a richly diverse group. Humor, love, and the joy of being alive are our only common denominators. . . . Through the expansion of my personality as a person with MS, I am firmly rooted in my past, fully living in the present, and planning a great future. I am at one with myself."

> Patricia Karn, artist and registered
> nurse (multiple sclerosis)

ON THE GOOD LIFE

"I believe very emphatically, very definitely, and very fervently that being alive is a beautiful experience, whether confronted by a physical disability or the normal process of aging."

> Carole Ann Parsons, social worker, consultant at
> a nursing home (respiratory polio quad)

"It is obvious that life has been very good to me and my physical disability has opened untold avenues of endeavor rather than creating insurmountable barriers."

> Tedde Kast Scharf (identified above)

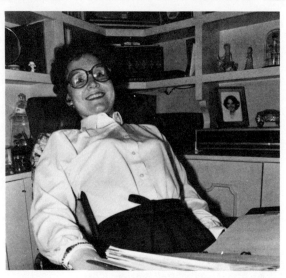

Cloir Jo Schnitz

FOR WOMEN ONLY

"I have spent most of my life saddled by a chest respirator and supported by a reclining wheelchair. This physical reality comprises a structural framework that occasionally creates annoying barriers, but that in no real way limits my spiritual, emotional, and intellectual development, except when I'm foolish enough to allow it. . . . Frankly, I think today's disabled woman has the advantages of choosing from both female worlds—she can select the role of feminine dependency because of her very real dependency, or she can opt to seek independence because she is a female in an age of women's struggle for equality, or she can find her own satisfactory balance between the two."

> Clare Jo Schnitz, part-time college tutor from Texas (respiratory polio quad)

"For all of us disabled women, life is difficult but it is necessary to try to make it less unpleasant and less difficult, for our own good and for those around us. How? By facing life with courage. . . . By insisting that our families do not limit us by overprotecting us. By doing the things we can do, no matter how small. By joining with other disabled persons for our common good. By requiring that society acknowledge our rights. . . . I know from my own experience that the drive to attain fulfillment sometimes fails before the limits that life places on us, but who today does not have limits? The daily struggle gives us honor, and poor is the person who has nothing to struggle for."

Gabriella Brimmer (identified above)

"I feel that what I do with my life as a woman is critical because I represent part of the mirror-image of disability as well as womanhood that is envisioned by society. I believe that it is essential for those of us who are disabled to overcome our fears, anxieties, and inhibitions and get out and live, so that our disabilities will become minimized and our examples will thus teach society that we are made of the same stuff as they. We are different only in that we can't move our arms and legs so well. In spite of the inconveniences of immobility, we laugh, we cry, and we make love. We have hopes, aspirations, successes, and failures. We go to school, work, take vacations, raise families, and make our contributions to society."

Bev Baer, Ohio social worker and
doctoral candidate in art education
(polio quad)

YOUR SPECIAL GIFT TO SOCIETY

The mother of a spina bifida child appeared recently on a Washington, D.C., television show along with her nine-year-old daughter, Nancy. The mother was talking about the special problems she and her daughter face every time they venture out, whether it be to go to a restaurant, a supermarket, or any other place. She explained the usual routines that were necessary—calling ahead, checking out accesses, arranging for transportation.

"We accept all this," she said, "but what really gets me down sometimes is that it seems that I must make everyone we meet feel *good* about Nancy. People's immediate reaction is one of pity. I believe they may want to offer help or sympathy, but they don't know how, so they look away in embarrassment."

The fact is that except for those who have had handicapped persons as members of their own families, people usually don't know how to treat the handicapped. The nonhandicapped are in the process of learning how to get along with their handicapped brothers and sisters who until recently have been too often hidden away.

Later in the television interview, Nancy's mother told about the public school her daughter attends. There were some special classes for the handicapped, but whenever possible they were mixed with the nonhandicapped. "Today's nonhandicapped children will not grow up with the embarrassments expressed by most of today's adults," Nancy's mother went on to say. "They are accepting handicapped classmates as being just the same as anyone else, except that they have special problems in one area or another."

This is indeed the attitude we all hope everyone will soon express toward handicapped people. The schools' new mainstreaming program is helping to bring this about. So is the new legislation prohibiting discrimination. You can make a contribution toward speeding this process in the following way.

Handicapped persons need to ask for help more than others. This may have been a source of embarrassment and frustration, but it is just this situation that provides you with an opportunity. More than most people in today's frantically busy world, you recognize the value of having friends, relatives, and neighbors who are sincerely interested in you and who want to help. In general our society seems to be losing a capacity for friendliness, neighborliness, loving-caring relationships, and even for good family relationships. By being in need of help, and especially by accepting needed help graciously, you are making a contribution no one else can make. You can be in the vanguard of those who lead us all to develop more cooperative, less antagonistic ways of relating to one another. When we do, we shall all have a happier, more peaceful world to live in.

We hope the statements quoted in this chapter can help you gain or regain a working philosophy of life that is meaningful.

As more and more of the handicapped view themselves as persons who can make contributions, so will it be. A relatively few people have changed the United States in so many positive ways. The handicapped people of this country numbering many millions—some visible, some not—will help to make our future a bright one. Their talents, love, and achievements will make the big difference as we move quickly toward the 21st century.

Appendix

This section contains lists that were referred to in several of the preceding chapters, as well as lists of additional general resources that may be helpful to you in pursuing your search for the right career and the right life-style.

NATIONAL VOLUNTARY HEALTH ASSOCIATIONS AND ORGANIZATIONS OF AND FOR HANDICAPPED PEOPLE

Blind
American Council of the Blind
1211 Connecticut Avenue, NW
Washington, DC 20036

American Foundation for the Blind
15 West 16th Street
New York, NY 10011

National Association for Visually Handicapped
22 West 21st Street
New York, NY 10010

National Federation for the Blind
1800 Johnston Street
Baltimore, MD 21230

Cerebral Palsy
United Cerebral Palsy Association
66 East 34th Street
New York, NY 10016

Deaf
Alexander Graham Bell Association for the Deaf
3417 Volta Place, NW
Washington, DC 20007

National Association of the Deaf
814 Thayer Avenue
Silver Spring, MD 20910

Deaf-Blind
National Association of the Deaf-Blind
2703 Forest Oak Circle
Norman, OK 73071

Dyslexia
The Orton Dyslexia Society
724 York Road
Baltimore, MD 21204

Emotionally Disturbed
Mental Health Association, National Headquarters
1800 North Kent Street
Arlington, VA 22209

Epilepsy
Epilepsy Foundation of America
1828 L Street, NW
Washington, DC 20036

Health Impairments
Asthma and Allergy Foundation of America
19 West 44th Street
New York, NY 10036

American Heart Association
7320 Greenville Avenue
Dallas, TX 75231

Cystic Fibrosis Foundation
6000 Executive Blvd.
Rockville, MD 20852

Juvenile Diabetes Foundation
60 Madison Avenue
New York, NY 10010-1550

National Hemophilia Foundation
19 West 34th Street
New York, NY 10001

National Kidney Foundation
2 Park Avenue
New York, NY 10016

Learning Disabilities
Association for Children with Learning Disabilities
4156 Library Road
Pittsburgh, PA 15234

Mental Retardation
American Association on Mental Deficiency
5101 Wisconsin Avenue, NW
Washington, DC 20016

Association for Retarded Citizens
2501 Avenue J
Arlington, TX 76011

Physically Handicapped
Arthritis Foundation
3400 Peachtree Road, NE
Atlanta, GA 30326

Muscular Dystrophy Association, Inc.
810 Seventh Avenue
New York, NY 10019

National Multiple Sclerosis Society
205 East 42nd Street
New York, NY 10017

National Spinal Cord Injury Foundation
369 Elliot Street
Newton Upper Falls, MA 02164

Spina Bifida Association of America
343 South Dearborn Street
Room 319
Chicago, IL 60604

National Amputation Foundation
12-45 150th Street
Whitestone, NY 11357

Speech Impairments
American Speech-Language-Hearing Association
10801 Rockville Pike
Rockville, MD 20852

All Disabilities
National Association of the Physically Handicapped
76 Elm Street
London, OH 43140

American Coalition of Citizens with Disabilities
1200 15th Street, NW, Suite 201
Washington, DC 20005

National Easter Seal Society
2023 West Ogden Avenue
Chicago, IL 60612

National Foundation–March of Dimes
1275 Mamaroneck Avenue
White Plains, NY 10605

REGIONAL OFFICES OF REHABILITATION SERVICES
OF THE DEPARTMENT OF HEALTH,
EDUCATION, AND WELFARE

Region I
(Conn., R.I., Maine,
N.H., Mass., Vt.)

Office of Rehabilitation Services
John F. Kennedy Federal Building
Government Center
Boston, MA 02203

Region II
(N.J., N.Y., V.I., P.R.)

Office of Rehabilitation Services
Jacob K. Javits Federal Building
26 Federal Plaza
New York, NY 10278

Region III
(Del., Pa., D.C. Va.,
Md., W. Va.)

Office of Rehabilitation Services
3535 Market Street
P.O. Box 13716
Philadelphia, PA 19101

Region IV
(Ala., Miss., Fla., N.C.,
Ga., S.C., Ky., Tenn.)

Office of Rehabilitation Services
101 Marietta Tower
Atlanta, GA 30323

Region V
(Ill., Minn., Ind., Ohio, Mich., Wisc.)

Office of Rehabilitation Services
300 South Wacker Drive
Chicago, IL 60606

Region VI
(Ark., Oka, La., Texas, N.M.)

Office of Rehabilitation Services
1200 Main Tower
Dallas, TX 75202

Region VII
(Iowa, Mo., Kans., Nebr.)

Office of Rehabilitation Services
601 East 12th Street
Kansas City, MO 64106

Region VIII
(Colo., S.D., Mont., Utah, N.D., Wyo.)

Office of Rehabilitation Services
19th and Stout Streets
Denver, CO 80294

Region IX
(Ariz., Nev., Calif., Guam, Hawaii, Trust Terr. of Pacific Islands,
Am. Samoa)

Office of Rehabilitation Services
Federal Office Building
United Nations Plaza
San Francisco, CA 94102

Region X
(Alaska, Ore., Id., Wash.)

Office of Rehabilitation Services
The Third and Broad Building
2901 Third Avenue
Seattle, WA 98121

OFFICES OF STATE VOCATIONAL
REHABILITATION AGENCIES

Alabama
Vocational Rehabilitation
State Board of Education
2129 East South Boulevard
Montgomery 36111-0586

Alaska
Office of Vocational Rehabilitation

Department of Education
Pouch F
(Alaska Office Building)
Juneau 99801

Arizona
Rehabilitation Service Administration
1300 West Washington
Phoenix 85007

Section of Rehabilitation for the Blind and Visually Impaired
4620 North 16th Street, Room 100
Phoenix 85016

Arkansas
Rehabilitation Service
Department of Rehabilitation Services
1401 Brookwood Drive
P.O. Box 3781
Little Rock 72203

California
Department of Rehabilitation
Health and Welfare Agency
830 K Street Mall
Sacramento 95814

Colorado
Division of Rehabilitation
State Department of Social Services
1575 Sherman Street
Denver 80203

Connecticut
Division of Vocational Rehabilitation
State Department of Education
600 Asylum Avenue
Hartford 06105

Board of Education and Services for the Blind
170 Ridge Road
Wethersfield 06109

Delaware
Division of Vocational Rehabilitation
Department of Labor
820 North French Street
Wilmington 19801

Bureau for the Visually Impaired
305 West 8th Street
Wilmington 19801

District of Columbia
Vocational Rehabilitation Division
Commission of Social Service
Office of Human Services
122 C St., NW
Washington 20001

Florida
Division of Vocational Rehabilitation
Dept. of Health and Rehabilitative Services
1309 Winewood Boulevard
Tallahassee 32301

Georgia
Division of Vocational Rehabilitation
Department of Human Resources
47 Trinity Avenue, SW
Atlanta 30334

Hawaii
Vocational Rehabilitation Division
Department of Social Services
P.O. Box 339
Honolulu 96809

Idaho
Vocational Rehabilitation Services
State Board of Education

1501 North McKinney
Boise 83704

Idaho Commission for the Blind
341 West Washington
Boise 83720

Illinois
Division of Vocational Rehabilitation
Department of Rehabilitation
623 East Adams Street
Springfield 62705

Indiana
Rehabilitation Services Board
Illinois Building
17 West Market Street
Indianapolis 46204

Iowa
Division of Rehabilitation Education and Services
State Board of Public Instruction
510 East 12th Street
Des Moines 50319

Commission for the Blind
4th and Keosauqua Way
Des Moines 50309

Kansas
Division of Vocational Rehabilitation
Dept. of Social and Rehabilitation Services
2700 West 6th Street
Smith-Wilson Building
Topeka 66606

Division of Services for the Blind
2700 West 6th Street
Biddle Building
Topeka 66606

Kentucky
Bureau of Rehabilitation Services
State Board of Education
Capital Plaza Office Tower
Frankfort 40601

Louisiana
Division of Vocational Rehabilitation
Department of Health and Human Resources
P.O. Box 44367
Baton Rouge 70804

Division for the Blind
Office of Human Development
1755 Flordia Boulevard
P.O. Box 28
Baton Rouge 70821

Maine
Bureau of Rehabilitation Services
State Human Services Office
State House
Augusta 04333

Maryland
Division of Vocational Rehabilitation
Department of Education
301 West Preston Street, Room 1004
Baltimore 21201

Massachusetts
Massachusetts Rehabilitation Commission
296 Boylston Street
Boston 02116

Commission for the Blind
110 Tremont Street
Boston 02108

Michigan
Vocational Rehabilitation Services
State Dept. of Education
P.O. Box 30010
Lansing 48909

Commission for the Blind
Department of Labor
309 North Washington
P.O. Box 30015
Lansing 48909

Minnesota
Division of Vocational Rehabilitation
State Department of Economic Security
390 North Robert Street
St. Paul 55101

Services for the Blind and Visually Handicapped
1745 University Avenue
St. Paul 55104

Mississippi
Division of Vocational Rehabilitation
Dept. of Education
1304 Walter Sillers State Office Building
P.O. Box 1698
Jackson 39205

Vocational Rehabilitation for the Blind
5455 Executive Place
P.O. Box 4872
Jackson 39216

Missouri
Division of Vocational Rehabilitation
State Board of Education
2401 East McCarty Street
Jefferson City 65102

Bureau for the Blind
State Office Building
Jefferson City 65103

Montana
Rehabilitative Services Division

Dept. of Social and Rehabilitation Services
P.O. Box 4210
Helena 59601

Division of Visual Services
Dept. of Social and Rehabilitation Services
111 Sanders
P.O. Box 4210
Helena 59601

Nebraska
Division of Rehabilitation Services
State Department of Education
301 Centennial Mall, 6th fl.
P.O. Box 94987
Lincoln, NE 68509

Nevada
Rehabilitation Divison
State Department of Human Resources
Capitol Complex
505 East King Street
Carson City 89710

Bureau of Services for the Blind
Capitol Complex
505 East King Street
Carson City 89710

New Hampshire
Vocational Rehabilitation Division
State Department of Education
410 State House Annex
Concord 03301

New Jersey
Divison of Vocational Rehabilitation
Department of Labor and Industry
Labor and Industry Building
John Fitch Plaza
Trenton 08625

Commission for the Blind and Visually Impaired
1100 Raymond Boulevard
Newark 07102

New Mexico
Vocational Rehabilitation
Dept. of Education
P.O. Box 1830
Santa Fe 87503

New York
Office of Vocational Rehabilitation
State Education Department
Education Building
Albany 12234

Commission for the Blind and Visually Impaired
40 Pearl Street
Albany 12243

North Carolina
Division of Vocational Rehabilitation Services
Department of Human Resources
620 North West Street
P.O. Box 26053
Raleigh 27611

Division of Services for the Blind
Department of Human Resources
309 Ashe Avenue
Raleigh 27606

North Dakota
Division of Vocational Rehabilitation
Social Services Board
1424 Century Avenue
State Capitol
Bismarck 58505

Ohio
Bureau of Vocational Rehabilitation
4656 Heaton Road
Columbus 43229

Oklahoma
Divison of Rehabilitative and Visual Services
State Department of Human Services
P.O. Box 25352
Oklahoma City 73125

Oregon
Vocational Rehabilitation Division
Dept. of Human Resources
2045 Silverton Rd., NE
Salem 97310

State Commission for the Blind
535 S.E. 12th Avenue
Portland 97214

Pennsylvania
Bureau of Vocational Rehabilitation
Labor and Industry Building
7th and Forster Streets
Harrisburg 17120

Bureau of Blindness and Visual Services
P.O. Box 2675
Harrisburg 17105

Puerto Rico
Vocational Rehabilitation
P.O. Box 1118
Hato Rey 00919

Rhode Island
Vocational Rehabilitation
Social and Rehabilitative Services
40 Fountain Street
Providence 02903

Division of Services for the Blind
46 Aborn Street
Providence 02903

South Carolina
Vocational Rehabilitation Dept.
Landmark Center, Room 301
3600 Forest Drive
P.O. Box 4945
Columbia 29240

Commission for the Blind
1430 Confederate Avenue
Columbia 29211

South Dakota
Division of Rehabilitation Services
Department of Vocational Rehabilitation
Richard F. Kneip Building
Pierre 57501

Tennessee
Division of Vocational Rehabilitation
Department of Education
1808 West End Building, Room 1400
Nashville 37203

The Alliance for the
   Blind and Visually Impaired
P,O. Box 41782
Memphis 38174

Texas
Texas Rehabilitation Commission
118 East Riverside Drive
Austin 78704

State Commission for the Blind
P.O. Box 12866
Austin 78711

Utah
Division of Rehabilitation Services
State Board of Education
250 East South Temple Street
Salt Lake City 84111

Vermont
Vocational Rehabilitation Division
Dept. of Social and Rehabilitation Services
103 South Main Street
Waterbury 05676

Division for the Blind and Visually Handicapped
103 South Main Street
Waterbury 05676

Virginia
Department of Rehabilitation Services
State Office of Human Resources
P.O. Box 11045
Richmond 23230

Virginia Department for the Visually Handicapped
397 Azalea Avenue
Richmond 23227

Virgin Islands
Department of Social Welfare
P.O. Box 550
Charlotte Amalie
St. Thomas 00801

Washington
Vocational Rehabilitation Services Division
Department of Social and Health Services
State Office Building
Mail Stop OB-44
Olympia 98504

State Department Services for the Blind
921 Lakeridge Drive, Room 202
Mail Stop FW-21
Olympia 98504

West Virginia
Division of Vocational Rehabilitation
State Board of Vocational Education
State Capitol Building
Charleston 25305

Wisconsin
Division of Vocational Rehabilitation
Department of Health and Social Services
State Office Building
1 West Wilson Street
Madison 53702

Wyoming
Division of Vocational Rehabilitation
State Department of Health and Social Services
Hathaway Building
Cheyenne 82002

REGIONAL OFFICES OF THE U.S. BUREAU OF LABOR STATISTICS

Region I
1603 JFK Federal Building
Government Center
Boston, MA 02203
Phone: (617) 223–6761

Region II
Suite 3400
1515 Broadway
New York, NY 10036
Phone: (212) 944-3121

Region III
3535 Market Street
P.O. Box 13309
Philadelphia, PA 19101
Phone: (215) 596–1154

Region IV
1371 Peachtree Street, NE
Atlanta, GA 30367
Phone: (404) 881-4418

Region V
9th Floor
Federal Office Building
230 South Dearborn Street
Chicago, IL 60604
Phone: (312) 353–1880

Region VI
Federal Building, Room 221
525 Griffin Street
Dallas, TX 75202
Phone: (214) 767-6971

Regions VII and VIII
911 Walnut Street
Kansas City, MO 64106
Phone: (816) 374–2481

Regions IX and X
450 Golden Gate Avenue
Box 36017
San Francisco, CA 94102
Phone: (415) 556–4678

STATE–FEDERAL EMPLOYMENT
SECURITY AGENCIES (Placement)*

Alabama
Department of Industrial Relations
649 Monroe Street
Montgomery, AL 36130

Alaska
Employment Security Division
Department of Labor
Fourth and Harris Streets
P.O. Box 1149
Juneau, AK 99811

Arizona
Department of Economic Security
1717 Jefferson
Phoenix, AZ 85007

Arkansas
Arkansas Employment Security Division
Department of Labor
P.O. Box 2981
Little Rock, AR 72203

California
Employment Development Department
800 Capital Mall
Sacramento, CA 95814

Colorado
Division of Employment and Training
Department of Labor and Employment
251 East 12th Avenue
Denver, CO 80203

Connecticut
Connecticut Employment Security Division
Connecticut Labor Dept.

---

* To find the agency in your area, consult your phone directory.

200 Foly Brook Boulevard
Wethersfield, CT 06109

Delaware
Department of Labor
820 North French Street
Wilmington, DE 19809

District of Columbia
Department of Employment Services
500 C Street, NW
Washington, DC 20001

District Unemployment Compensation Board
Sixth and Pennsylvania Avenue, NW
Washington, DC 20001

Florida
Division of Employment Security
Department of Labor and Employment Security
201 Caldwell Building
Tallahassee, FL 32304

Georgia
Employment Security Agency
Department of Labor
State Labor Building
254 Washington Street, SW
Atlanta, GA 30334

Guam
Department of Labor
Government of Guam
P.O. Box 23548 GMF
Agana, Guam 96921

Hawaii
Department of Labor and Industrial Relations
830 Punchbowl Street
Honolulu, HA 96813
(808) 548-3150

Idaho
Department of Employment
317 Main Street
Boise, ID 83735

Illinois
Bureau of Employment Security
Department of Labor
910 South Michigan Avenue
Chicago, IL 60605

Indiana
Employment Security Division
10 North Senate Avenue
Indianapolis, IN 46204

Iowa
Iowa Department of Job Service
1000 East Grand Avenue
Des Moines, IA 50319

Kansas
Division of Employment
Department of Human Resources
401 Topeka Avenue
Topeka, Kansas 66603

Kentucky
Bureau of Manpower Services
Department of Human Resources
275 East Main Street
Frankfort, KY 40621

Louisiana
Office of Employment Security
Department of Labor
P.O. Box 44094
Baton Rouge, LA 70804

Maine
Bureau of Employment Security
Department of Manpower Affairs
20 Union Street
P.O. Box 309
Augusta, ME 04330

Maryland
Department of Employment Training
1100 North Eutaw Street
Baltimore, MD 21201

Massachusetts
Division of Employment Security
Charles F. Hurley Employment Sec. Building
Boston, MA 02114

Michigan
Employment Security Commission
7310 Woodward Avenue
Detroit, MI 48202

Minnesota
Department of Economic Security
390 North Robert Street
St. Paul, MN 55101

Mississippi
Employment Commission
1520 West Capitol Street
P.O. Box 1699
Jackson, MS 39205

Missouri
Division of Employment Security
Department of Labor and Industrial Relations
421 East Dunkin Street
P.O. Box 59
Jefferson City, MO. 65101

Montana
Employment Security Division
Department of Labor and Industry
P.O. Box 1728
Helena, MT 59601

Nebraska
Division of Employment
Department of Labor
550 South 16th Street
Lincoln, NB 68509

Nevada
Employment Security Department
500 East Third Street
Carson City, NV 89713

New Hampshire
Department of Employment Security
32 South Main Street, Room 204
Concord, NH 03301

New Jersey
Division of Employment Services
Department of Labor and Industry
John Fitch Plaza
Trenton, NJ 08625

New Mexico
Employment Security Department
P.O. Box 1928
Alnuquerque, NM 87103

New York
Department of Labor
State Campus, Bldg. #12
Albany, NY 12240

North Carolina
Employment Security Commission

200 West Jones Street
P.O. Box 25903
Raleigh, NC 27611

North Dakota
Job Service North Dakota
1000 East Divide Avenue
P.O. Box 1537
Bismarck, ND 58505

Ohio
Bureau of Employment Services
145 South Front Street
Columbus, OH 43216

Oklahoma
Employment Security Commission
200 Will Rogers Memorial Office Building
Oklahoma City, OK 73105

Oregon
Employment Division
Department of Human Resources
875 Union St., NE
Salem, OR 97311

Pennsylvania
Office of Employment Security
Department of Labor and Industry
1720 Labor and Industry Building
Harrisburg, PA 17121

Puerto Rico
Bureau of Employment Security
Department of Labor and Human Resources
505 Munoz Rivera Avenue
Hato Rey, PR 00918

Rhode Island
Dept. of Employment Security

24 Mason Street
Providence, RI 02903

South Carolina
Employment Security Commission
1550 Gadsden Street
P.O. Box 995
Columbia, SC 29202

South Dakota
Department of Labor
Capitol Lake Plaza
Pierre, SD 57501

Tennessee
Department of Employment Security
Cordell Hull State Office Building
Nashville, TN 37219

Texas
Employment Commission
638 TEC Bldg.
15th and Congress Avenue
Austin, TX 78778

Utah
Department of Employment Security
174 Social Hall Avenue
P.O. Box 11249
Salt Lake City, UT 84147

Vermont
Department of Employment Security
5 Green Mountain Drive
P.O. Box 488
Montpelier, VT 05602

Virginia
Virginia Employment Commission
Department of Labor and Industry

703 East Main Street
P.O. Box 1358
Richmond, VA 23211

Virgin Islands
Employment Security Agency
P.O. Box 706
Christiansted
St. Croix, VI 00820

Washington
Employment Security Department
212 Maple Park
Olympia, WA 98504

West Virginia
Dept. of Employment Security
112 California Avenue
Charleston, WV 25305

Wisconsin
Job Service Wisconsin
Department of Industry, Labor and Human Relations
201 East Washington Avenue
Madison, WI 53707

Wyoming
Employment Security Commission
Center and Midwest Streets
Casper, WY 82601

U.S. OFFICE OF PERSONNEL MANAGEMENT
(formerly Civil Service Commission)

FEDERAL JOB INFORMATION CENTERS

Note: Many of the more populated states have more than one center. We have included only one per state. To find the one nearest you, call the office given for a referral, or consult the local phone book under the U.S. Government section.

Alabama
Southerland Building
806 Governors Drive, SW
Huntsville, AL 35801
(205) 453-5070

Alaska
Federal Building
701 C Street, Box 22
Anchorage, AK 99513
(907) 271-5821

Arizona
U.S. Postal Service Building
522 North Central Building
Phoenix, AZ 85004
(602) 261-4736

Arkansas
Federal Building, Third Floor
700 West Capitol Avenue
Little Rock, AR 72201
(501) 378-5842

California
1029 J Street, Room 202
Sacramento, CA 95814
(916) 440-3441

Colorado
12345 West Alameda Parkway
P.O. Box 25167
Denver, CO 80225
(303) 837-3509

Connecticut
Federal Building, Room 613

450 Main Street
Hartford, CT 06103
(203) 722-3096

Delaware
800 West Fourth Street
Adams Four Shopping Plaza
Suite 102
Wilmington, DE 19801
(302) 571-2745

District of Columbia
1900 E Street, NW
Washington, DC 20415
(202) 737-9616

Florida
Federal Building and U.S. Courthouse
80 North Hughey Ave.
Orlando, FL 32801
(305) 420-6148

Georgia
Richard B. Russell Federal Building,
   9th Floor
75 Spring Street, SW
Atlanta, GA 30303
(404) 221–4315

Hawaii
Federal Building, Room 1310
300 Ala Moana Boulevard
Honolulu, HA 96850
(808) 546-8600

Idaho
Call the Seattle Office
(206) 442-4365

Illinois
55 East Jackson, Room 1401
Chicago, IL 60604
(312) 353-5136

Indiana
46 East Ohio Street
Room 124
Indianapolis, IN 46204
(317 269-7161

Iowa
210 Walnut Street
Room 191
Des Moines, IA 50309
(515) 284-4545

Kansas
One-Twenty Building, Room 101
120 South Market Street
Wichita, KS 67202
(316) 269-6106

Kentucky
Call the Memphis Office
(901) 521-3956

Louisiana
F. Edward Hebert Building
610 South Street, Room 849
New Orleans, LA 70130
(504) 589-2764

Maine
Federal Building
Augusta, ME 04330
(800) 452-8732

Maryland
Garmatz Federal Building
101 West Lombard Street
Baltimore, MD 21201
(301) 962-3822

Massachusetts
3 Center Plaza
Boston, MA 02108
(617) 223-2571

Michigan
477 Michigan Avenue
Room 565
Detroit, MI 48226
(313) 226-6950

Minnesota
Federal Building
Ft. Snelling
Twin Cities, MN 55111
(612) 725-4430

Mississippi
100 West Capitol Street
Suite 335
Jackson, MS 39260
(601) 960-4585

Missouri
Federal Building, Room 134
601 East 12th Street
Kansas City, MO 64106
(816) 374-5702

Montana
Call the Seattle Office
(206) 442-4365

Nebraska
U.S. Courthouse and Post Office
   Building
Room 1010
215 North 17th Street
Omaha, NB 68102
(402) 221-3815

Nevada
Call the Sacramento Office
(916) 440-3441

New Hampshire
Federal Building, Room 104
80 Daniel Street
Portsmouth, NH 03801
(603) 436-7720, ext. 762

New Jersey
Federal Building
970 Broad Street
Newark, NJ 07102
(201) 645-3673

New Mexico
Federal Building
421 Gold Avenue, SW
Albuquerque, NM 87102
(505) 766-5583

New York
Jacob K. Javits Federal Building
26 Federal Plaza
New York, NY 10278
(212) 264-0422

North Carolina
Federal Building
310 New Bern
Raleigh, NC 27611
(919) 856-4361

North Dakota
Call the Denver Office
(303) 236-4163

Ohio
Federal Building

200 West 2nd Street
Dayton, OH 45402
(513) 225-2720

Oklahoma
200 N.W. Fifth Street, Room 205
Oklahoma City, OK 73102
(405) 231-4948

Oregon
Federal Building
1220 S.W. Third Street
Portland, OR 97204
(503) 221-3141

Pennsylvania
Federal Building, Room 168
Harrisburg, PA 17108
(717) 782-4494

Puerto Rico
Federico Degetau Federal Building
Charlos E. Chardon Street
Hato Rey, PR 00918
(809) 753-4209

Rhode Island
John O. Pastori Federal Building
    Room 310
Kennedy Plaza
Providence, RI 02903
(401) 528-5251

South Carolina
Federal Building
334 Meeting Street
Charleston, SC 29403
(803) 724-4328

South Dakota
Call the Denver Office
(303) 236-4164

Tennessee
100 North Main Street
Suite 312
Memphis, TN 38103
(901) 521-3956

Texas
1100 Commerce Street
Room 6B4
Dallas, TX 75242
(214) 767-8035

Utah
Call the Denver Office
(303) 236-4165

Vermont
Call the Portsmith Office
(603) 431-7115

Virginia
Federal Building
Room 220

200 Granby Mall
Norfolk, VA 23510
(804) 441-3355

Washington
Federal Building
915 Second Avenue
Seattle, WA 98174
(206) 442-4365

West Virginia
Federal Building
500 Quarrier Street
Charleston, WV 25301
(304) 343–6181, ext. 226

Wisconsin
Call the Chicago Office
(312) 353-5136

Wyoming
Call the Denver Office
(303) 236-3432

Index

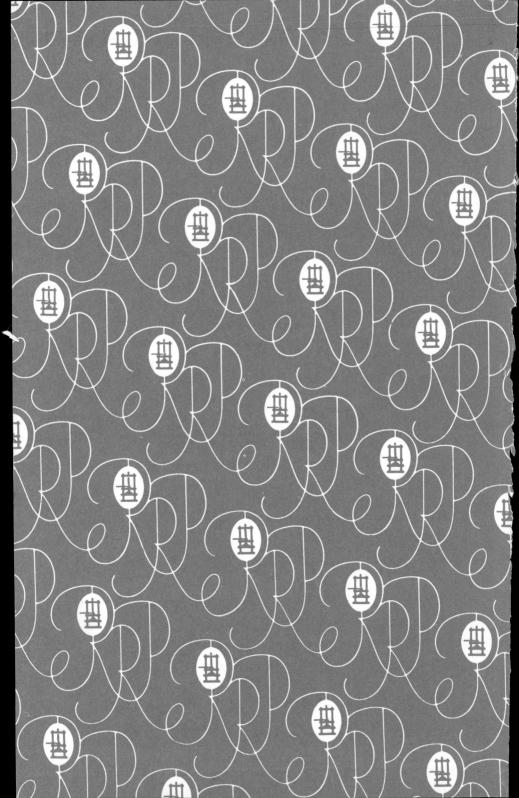